Conquering Diverticulitis And Diverticulosis

NATURAL REMEDIES AND HOLISTIC HEALING FOR DIGESTIVE HEATH

JULIA MARTIN

Copyright

No part of this book should be copied, reproduced without the author's permission @2024 Conquering Diverticulitis And Diverticulosis by Julia Martin.

TABLE OF CONTENTS

Copyright 2

TABLE OF CONTENTS 3

Introduction 6

    Purpose of the book 8

    Importance of natural remedies and holistic healing 11

Chapter 1 14

Understanding Diverticulitis and Diverticulosis 14

    Causes and Risk Factors 15

    Dietary influences 19

    Lifestyle factors 22

    Age-related changes 26

Chapter 2 30

Diverticulitis vs Diverticulosis 30

    Diagnosis 32

    Common symptoms of diverticulosis and diverticulitis 33

    Managing Symptoms 36

    Importance of early detection 40

Chapter 3 43

Conventional Treatments 43

    Overview of medical treatments 44

    Medications and their uses 48

    Surgical options and when they are necessary 52

Long-term strategies for maintaining digestive health _____ 56

Chapter 4 _____ 61
Dietary Modifications _____ 61
Importance of a high-fiber diet _____ 64
Foods to avoid and foods to include _____ 67
Sample meal plans and recipes _____ 72
Hydration and its role in digestive health _____ 80

Chapter 5 _____ 85
Natural Remedies and Supplements _____ 85
Herbal remedies and their benefits _____ 87
Probiotics and prebiotics _____ 92
Vitamins and minerals essential for gut health _____ 98

Chapter 6 _____ 105
Lifestyle Changes for Better Digestive Health _____ 105
Exercise and physical activity _____ 107
Stress management techniques _____ 112
How to prevent diverticulosis from progressing to diverticulitis _____ 116
Regular medical check-ups and monitoring _____ 119

Chapter 7 _____ 121
Holistic Approaches to Healing _____ 121
Integrative medicine and its role in treatment _____ 122
Mind-body connection and practices _____ 126
Acupuncture and other alternative therapies _____ 130

Chapter 8 _____ *135*
Living with Diverticulitis and Diverticulosis _____ ***135***
   Managing daily life with diverticular disease _____ **136**
   Coping strategies and support systems _____ **140**
Conclusion _____ ***146***

Introduction

Diverticulitis and diverticulosis are increasingly common digestive disorders that affect millions of people worldwide. While these conditions are often dismissed as minor issues, they can significantly impact one's quality of life, leading to severe discomfort, pain, and complications if left unmanaged. Understanding and effectively managing these conditions is crucial for maintaining overall digestive health and well-being.

Diverticulosis occurs when small pouches, known as diverticula, form in the walls of the colon. These pouches are usually asymptomatic but can lead to diverticulitis when they become inflamed or infected. Symptoms of diverticulitis can range from mild abdominal pain to severe complications such as abscesses, perforations, and even life-threatening infections. The progression from diverticulosis to diverticulitis highlights the importance of early detection and proactive management.

Conventional treatments for diverticulitis often involve antibiotics, pain management, and, in severe cases, surgery. While these treatments can be effective, they do not address the underlying causes or provide long-term solutions. Moreover, the overuse of antibiotics can lead to resistance and other adverse effects. This is where natural remedies and holistic approaches come into play.

In "Healing Diverticulitis and Diverticulosis: Natural Remedies for Digestive Health," we will explore a comprehensive range of strategies to manage and prevent these conditions. From dietary modifications and herbal supplements to lifestyle changes and mind-body practices, this book provides practical and effective solutions to support digestive health naturally.

Our goal is to empower you with knowledge and tools to take control of your health. You will learn about the importance of a high-fibre diet, the benefits of probiotics, and the role of stress management in maintaining a healthy gut. We will also delve into the latest research and emerging treatments, offering hope and insight into the future of diverticular disease management.

Whether you have been recently diagnosed, are looking for preventive measures, or are seeking alternative treatments, this book is your guide to understanding and overcoming diverticulitis and diverticulosis. Through natural remedies and holistic healing, you can achieve better digestive health and improve your overall quality of life.

Purpose of the book

The purpose of "Healing Diverticulitis and Diverticulosis: Natural Remedies for Digestive Health" is to provide a comprehensive guide that empowers individuals to understand, manage, and prevent diverticular diseases through natural and holistic approaches. This book aims to bridge the gap between conventional medical treatments and alternative healing methods, offering readers a well-rounded perspective on maintaining digestive health.

Diverticulitis and diverticulosis are often misunderstood and under-recognized conditions that can significantly impact one's quality of life. Many people suffer in silence, unsure of how to manage their symptoms or prevent flare-ups effectively. This book seeks to demystify these conditions by providing clear, accurate, and accessible information on their causes, symptoms, and treatments.

One of the primary goals of this book is to emphasize the importance of natural remedies and lifestyle changes in managing diverticular diseases. While conventional treatments such as antibiotics and surgery can be effective, they often address only the symptoms rather than the underlying causes. By exploring dietary modifications, herbal supplements, probiotics, and stress management techniques, this book offers readers practical tools to support their digestive health from the inside out.

Another key purpose of this book is to highlight the role of diet in preventing and managing diverticular diseases. Many people are unaware of the profound impact that their dietary choices can have on their digestive health. Through detailed guidance on high-fibre foods, hydration, and balanced nutrition, readers will learn how to make informed dietary decisions that promote gut health and prevent complications.

In addition to dietary advice, this book delves into the benefits of holistic practices such as yoga, meditation, and acupuncture. These mind-body approaches can play a crucial role in reducing stress, improving digestion, and enhancing overall well-being. By integrating these practices into their daily lives, readers can achieve a more balanced and healthy lifestyle.

This book also aims to provide hope and support to those living with diverticulitis and diverticulosis. Personal stories and testimonials from individuals who have successfully managed their conditions offer inspiration and practical insights. Moreover, the latest research and emerging treatments discussed in the book provide readers with a glimpse into the future of diverticular disease management.

Ultimately, the purpose of "Healing Diverticulitis and Diverticulosis: Natural Remedies for Digestive Health" is to empower readers to take control of their digestive health through natural and holistic means. By understanding their condition and exploring alternative treatments, readers can achieve better health outcomes and improve their overall quality of life.

Importance of natural remedies and holistic healing

Natural remedies and holistic healing play a crucial role in managing diverticulitis and diverticulosis, offering a more comprehensive approach to health and wellness compared to conventional treatments alone. The importance of these methods lies in their ability to address the root causes of digestive issues, promote overall gut health, and enhance the body's natural healing processes.

Addressing Root Causes:
Conventional treatments for diverticular diseases often focus on alleviating symptoms rather than addressing underlying factors. Natural remedies, such as dietary modifications and herbal supplements, aim to tackle the root causes, such as inflammation and poor gut health. By improving digestion and reducing inflammation, these remedies can help prevent the recurrence of symptoms and complications.

Promoting Gut Health:
A high-fibre diet, rich in fruits, vegetables, and whole grains, is fundamental in managing

diverticular diseases. Fibre helps regulate bowel movements, reduce pressure in the colon, and prevent the formation of diverticula. Probiotics, beneficial bacteria found in fermented foods and supplements, also play a vital role in maintaining a healthy gut microbiome, which is essential for overall digestive health.

Enhancing Natural Healing:
Holistic practices, such as stress management techniques, yoga, and meditation, contribute to overall well-being by reducing stress levels, which can exacerbate digestive issues. Chronic stress negatively impacts gut health by altering the gut-brain axis, leading to inflammation and weakened immune responses. Incorporating these practices can improve mental health and, in turn, support a healthier digestive system.

Reducing Dependency on Medications:
Natural remedies can reduce the need for long-term use of medications, which often come with side effects and potential complications. For instance, overuse of antibiotics can lead to antibiotic resistance and disrupt the balance of gut bacteria. By adopting natural and holistic approaches,

individuals can minimize these risks and promote sustainable health.

In summary, the importance of natural remedies and holistic healing in managing diverticulitis and diverticulosis lies in their ability to provide a balanced, comprehensive approach to health. By addressing root causes, promoting gut health, enhancing natural healing, and reducing dependency on medications, these methods offer a pathway to improved digestive health and overall well-being.

Chapter 1

Understanding Diverticulitis and Diverticulosis

Diverticulitis and diverticulosis are closely related conditions that affect the colon, part of the digestive system. Diverticulosis occurs when small pouches, known as diverticula, form in the walls of the colon. This condition is often asymptomatic and is typically discovered during routine colonoscopies. However, if these pouches become inflamed or infected, the condition progresses to diverticulitis.

Diverticulitis can cause a range of symptoms, from mild abdominal pain to severe complications such as abscesses, perforations, and infections. Common symptoms include sharp pain in the lower left abdomen, fever, nausea, and changes in bowel habits. The severity of these symptoms can vary, and in some cases, diverticulitis can lead to life-threatening complications if not properly managed.

Understanding the differences between diverticulosis and diverticulitis is crucial for effective management and prevention. While diverticulosis can often be managed with dietary and lifestyle changes to prevent progression, diverticulitis may require medical intervention, including antibiotics or surgery in severe cases.

This chapter provides a foundational understanding of these conditions, their development, and their impact on the digestive system. By recognizing the signs and knowing how to manage both diverticulosis and diverticulitis, individuals can take proactive steps towards better digestive health.

Causes and Risk Factors

Understanding the causes and risk factors for diverticulosis and diverticulitis is essential for effective prevention and management. While the exact causes are not entirely understood, several contributing factors have been identified.

Dietary Influences

A low-fibre diet is one of the most significant risk factors for developing diverticulosis and diverticulitis. Fibre helps to soften stool and promote regular bowel movements, reducing pressure in the colon. Diets high in refined carbohydrates, red meat, and low in fruits, vegetables, and whole grains can lead to constipation and increased pressure on the colon walls, contributing to the formation of diverticula.

Age

The prevalence of diverticulosis increases with age. As people get older, the walls of the colon may weaken, making it easier for diverticula to form. It's estimated that about half of people over the age of 60 have diverticulosis.

Lifestyle Factors

Certain lifestyle factors, such as physical inactivity, obesity, and smoking, can increase the risk of diverticular diseases. Lack of exercise can lead to slower bowel movements and increased pressure on the colon. Obesity, particularly abdominal obesity, is linked to higher pressure within the colon, contributing to the formation of diverticula. Smoking has been associated with a higher risk of complications from diverticulitis.

Genetic Predisposition

There is evidence to suggest that genetics play a role in the development of diverticulosis and diverticulitis. If a close family member has diverticular disease, you may be at an increased risk. Studies have shown that certain genetic markers are associated with an increased susceptibility to these conditions.

Chronic Constipation

Chronic constipation can lead to increased pressure within the colon, promoting the formation of diverticula. Straining during bowel movements can exacerbate this pressure, making it more likely for diverticulosis to develop and progress to diverticulitis.

Connective Tissue Disorders

Conditions that affect the connective tissues, such as Ehlers-Danlos syndrome or Marian syndrome, can also increase the risk of developing diverticula. These disorders can cause weakness in the colon walls, making them more susceptible to bulging and forming pouches.

Use of Certain Medications

The use of nonsteroidal anti-inflammatory drugs (NSAIDs), steroids, and opioids has been linked to an increased risk of diverticulitis. These medications can affect the integrity of the colon lining, making it more susceptible to inflammation and infection.

Previous Episodes of Diverticulitis

Having had diverticulitis once increases the risk of recurrence. Each subsequent episode can lead to further complications, such as abscesses, fistulas, or perforations in the colon.

The development of diverticulosis and diverticulitis is influenced by a combination of dietary habits, age, lifestyle factors, genetics, chronic constipation, connective tissue disorders, medication use, and previous episodes of diverticulitis. Understanding these risk factors can help individuals take proactive measures to prevent the onset and progression of these conditions. By adopting a high-fibre diet, maintaining a healthy lifestyle, and being aware of genetic predispositions, individuals can reduce their risk and manage their digestive health more effectively.

Dietary influences

Diet plays a crucial role in the development and management of diverticulosis and diverticulitis. A poor diet, particularly one low in fibre, is one of the most significant risk factors for these conditions.

Low-Fibre Diet:
A diet low in fibre is strongly associated with the formation of diverticula, which characterizes diverticulosis. Fibre adds bulk to stool and helps it pass more easily through the digestive tract. Without adequate fibre, stool becomes harder and more difficult to move, increasing pressure in the colon. This pressure can cause weak spots in the colon wall to bulge out, forming diverticula. Consistently consuming low-fibre foods, such as refined grains, processed foods, and low-fibre snacks, contributes to this problem.

Refined Carbohydrates:
Foods high in refined carbohydrates, such as white bread, pastries, and sugary snacks, can contribute to the development of diverticular disease. These

foods often lack essential nutrients and fibre, leading to poor bowel function and increased risk of constipation. The lack of fibre in these foods means they pass through the digestive system more slowly, increasing the time stool remains in the colon and the pressure exerted on the colon walls.

Red Meat:
A diet high in red meat, particularly processed meats, is linked to an increased risk of diverticulitis. Red meat can contribute to inflammation in the body, including the colon. Additionally, a diet rich in red meat often means lower intake of fibre-rich foods, exacerbating the risk.

Lack of Fruits and Vegetables:
Fruits and vegetables are excellent sources of dietary fibre, vitamins, and minerals. A diet lacking in these foods can lead to insufficient fibre intake, contributing to the formation of diverticula. Moreover, fruits and vegetables provide antioxidants and anti-inflammatory compounds that help maintain overall gut health and reduce the risk of inflammation.

Hydration:
Adequate hydration is essential for

maintaining healthy bowel function. Water helps soften stool, making it easier to pass and reducing the risk of constipation. Without sufficient fluid intake, stool can become hard and dry, increasing the risk of diverticular disease. It's crucial to drink plenty of water, especially when increasing fibre intake, to help fibre work effectively.

Probiotics and Fermented Foods:
Probiotics, found in fermented foods like yogurt, kefir, sauerkraut, and kimchi, can help maintain a healthy balance of gut bacteria. A healthy gut microbiome is crucial for preventing inflammation and maintaining overall digestive health. Including these foods in the diet can support gut health and reduce the risk of diverticulitis flare-ups.

High-Fibre Foods:
To reduce the risk of diverticulosis and manage diverticulitis, it is essential to incorporate high-fibre foods into the diet. Foods such as whole grains, legumes, fruits, vegetables, nuts, and seeds provide the necessary fibre to promote regular bowel movements and reduce colon pressure. Gradually increasing fibre intake can help the digestive system adjust and prevent discomfort.

Dietary choices significantly impact the risk of developing diverticulosis and diverticulitis. A diet low in fibre, high in refined carbohydrates, and rich in red meat can increase the likelihood of these conditions. Conversely, a diet high in fibre, rich in fruits and vegetables, and supported by adequate hydration and probiotic intake can help prevent diverticular disease and manage its symptoms effectively. Making informed dietary choices is a fundamental step toward better digestive health and overall well-being.

Lifestyle factors

Lifestyle factors play a significant role in the development and management of diverticulosis and diverticulitis. Certain habits and behaviour's can increase the risk of these conditions, while others can help prevent them and improve overall digestive health.

Physical Inactivity:
A sedentary lifestyle is a major risk factor for diverticular diseases. Regular physical activity helps stimulate bowel movements and reduces the pressure within the colon. Lack of exercise can lead

to slower transit times, increasing the risk of constipation and the formation of diverticula. Incorporating regular exercise, such as walking, jogging, or strength training, can improve gut motility and overall digestive health.

Obesity:
Excess body weight, particularly abdominal obesity, is associated with an increased risk of diverticulosis and diverticulitis. Excess fat in the abdominal area can increase pressure on the colon, leading to the formation of diverticula. Maintaining a healthy weight through diet and exercise can help reduce this risk.

Smoking:
Smoking is linked to numerous health issues, including an increased risk of complications from diverticulitis. Nicotine and other chemicals in cigarettes can affect the integrity of the colon lining and promote inflammation. Quitting smoking can significantly reduce the risk of diverticulitis and improve overall health.

Alcohol Consumption:
Excessive alcohol consumption can irritate the digestive tract and contribute to inflammation. While

moderate alcohol consumption may not have a significant impact, heavy drinking can increase the risk of diverticulitis flare-ups. Limiting alcohol intake can help maintain digestive health and reduce the risk of complications.

Stress:
Chronic stress can negatively impact the digestive system. The gut-brain axis, which links the emotional and cognitive centres of the brain with peripheral intestinal functions, can be disrupted by stress. This disruption can lead to inflammation, changes in gut motility, and an increased risk of diverticulitis. Stress management techniques, such as yoga, meditation, and mindfulness, can help reduce stress and improve gut health.

Inadequate Sleep:
Poor sleep quality and insufficient sleep can negatively affect overall health, including digestive health. Sleep is essential for the body's repair and maintenance processes. Chronic sleep deprivation can lead to hormonal imbalances and increased inflammation, raising the risk of diverticular diseases. Prioritizing good sleep hygiene and ensuring adequate rest can support overall well-being and digestive health.

Hydration:
Adequate hydration is vital for healthy bowel function. Drinking enough water helps soften stool and promotes regular bowel movements, reducing the risk of constipation and diverticula formation. It's essential to drink plenty of fluids throughout the day, especially when consuming a high-fibre diet.

Dietary Habits:
While diet was discussed earlier, lifestyle habits related to eating are also crucial. Eating meals at regular intervals, chewing food thoroughly, and avoiding excessive consumption of processed foods can positively impact digestive health. Mindful eating practices can aid digestion and reduce the risk of diverticular disease.

Lifestyle factors such as physical inactivity, obesity, smoking, alcohol consumption, stress, inadequate sleep, hydration, and dietary habits play a significant role in the development and management of diverticulosis and diverticulitis. By adopting a healthy and active lifestyle, individuals can reduce their risk and promote better digestive health. Making informed choices about exercise, stress management, sleep, and hydration can help prevent diverticular diseases and improve overall well-being.

Age-related changes

Age is a significant risk factor for the development of diverticulosis and diverticulitis. As people age, several physiological changes occur that can increase the likelihood of these conditions.

Colon Wall Weakening:
One of the primary age-related changes is the weakening of the colon walls. Over time, the connective tissues that support the colon can lose their strength and elasticity, making it easier for small pouches, or diverticula, to form. This weakening is a natural part of the aging process and is more pronounced in older adults.

Decreased Fibre Intake:
Many older adults may experience changes in their dietary habits, often consuming less fibre due to changes in appetite, dental issues, or difficulty in preparing high-fibre meals. A lower intake of dietary fibre can lead to constipation and increased

pressure in the colon, contributing to the formation of diverticula.

Slower Bowel Movements:
Aging can lead to a slowdown in bowel motility. The muscles in the digestive tract may become less efficient, resulting in slower transit times for food and waste. This can cause constipation and increase the risk of diverticula formation due to prolonged pressure on the colon walls.

Changes in Gut Microbiota:
The composition of gut microbiota changes with age, potentially impacting overall digestive health. A less diverse microbiota can lead to an imbalance that promotes inflammation and weakens the colon walls. Maintaining a healthy balance of gut bacteria through diet and probiotics can help mitigate these effects.

Increased Medication Use:
Older adults are often prescribed multiple medications for various health conditions. Some medications, such as nonsteroidal anti-inflammatory drugs (NSAIDs), steroids, and certain pain relievers, can increase the risk of diverticulitis by affecting the

integrity of the colon lining and promoting inflammation.

Reduced Physical Activity:
Physical activity tends to decrease with age, contributing to slower bowel movements and increased risk of constipation. Regular exercise is essential for maintaining healthy bowel function and reducing the pressure on the colon. Encouraging older adults to engage in appropriate physical activities can help mitigate this risk.

Comorbidities:
As people age, they are more likely to develop other health conditions, such as diabetes, cardiovascular disease, and hypertension. These comorbidities can indirectly affect digestive health by influencing diet, physical activity levels, and overall bodily functions.

Weakened Immune System:
Aging is associated with a gradual decline in immune function, which can affect the body's ability to fight off infections, including those that may affect the colon. A weakened immune system can increase the susceptibility to infections that may lead to diverticulitis.

Age-related changes significantly contribute to the risk of developing diverticulosis and diverticulitis. These changes include weakening of the colon walls, decreased fibre intake, slower bowel movements, alterations in gut microbiota, increased medication use, reduced physical activity, the presence of comorbidities, and a weakened immune system. Understanding these age-related factors can help in developing targeted strategies to prevent and manage diverticular diseases in older adults, promoting better digestive health and overall well-being.

Chapter 2

Diverticulitis vs Diverticulosis

Understanding the distinction between diverticulitis and diverticulosis is crucial for effective management and treatment. Though these terms are often used interchangeably, they refer to different stages and conditions within the spectrum of diverticular disease.

Diverticulosis:
Diverticulosis is a condition characterized by the presence of small pouches, or diverticula, that protrude from the walls of the colon. These pouches form due to increased pressure within the colon, often resulting from a low-fibre diet or chronic constipation. Diverticulosis is typically asymptomatic and is usually discovered incidentally during routine colonoscopies or imaging tests. While many individuals with diverticulosis may never experience symptoms, it remains essential to manage the condition through dietary and lifestyle changes to prevent progression.

Diverticulitis:

Diverticulitis occurs when one or more of the diverticula become inflamed or infected. This inflammation can cause a range of symptoms, from mild abdominal pain and discomfort to severe complications like abscesses, perforations, and peritonitis. Common symptoms of diverticulitis include sharp pain, typically in the lower left abdomen, fever, nausea, and changes in bowel habits such as constipation or diarrhoea. Diverticulitis can be acute or chronic, with recurrent episodes leading to more significant complications over time.

Key Differences:

The primary difference between diverticulosis and diverticulitis is the presence of inflammation or infection. Diverticulosis refers to the mere existence of diverticula without inflammation, while diverticulitis involves active inflammation and infection. Management strategies also differ: diverticulosis is generally managed through preventive measures such as a high-fibre diet, adequate hydration, and regular exercise. In contrast, diverticulitis often requires medical treatment, including antibiotics and, in severe cases, surgery.

Recognizing the differences between diverticulosis and diverticulitis is vital for appropriate management and treatment. While diverticulosis can often be managed with lifestyle changes, diverticulitis requires prompt medical attention to address inflammation and prevent complications.

Diagnosis

Diagnosing diverticulosis and diverticulitis involves a combination of patient history, physical examination, and diagnostic tests. For diverticulosis, which is often asymptomatic, the condition is typically discovered incidentally during routine screenings like colonoscopies or imaging studies conducted for other reasons.

Physical Examination:
During a physical exam, a doctor may check for abdominal tenderness or pain, which can indicate inflammation or infection, particularly in the case of diverticulitis.

Diagnostic Tests:

- Colonoscopy: This procedure involves inserting a flexible tube with a camera into the colon to visualize diverticula directly.
- CT Scan: A CT scan is the preferred imaging method for diagnosing diverticulitis, as it can detect inflammation, abscesses, and other complications.
- Blood Tests: Blood tests can reveal signs of infection or inflammation, such as elevated white blood cell counts.
- Ultrasound or MRI: In some cases, these imaging tests may be used to provide additional information or if a CT scan is not suitable.

Early and accurate diagnosis is crucial for effective management and treatment of both conditions.

Common symptoms of diverticulosis and diverticulitis

Understanding the symptoms of diverticulosis and diverticulitis is essential for early identification and management of these conditions. While they share a common root in the formation of diverticula, the symptoms and their severity differ significantly.

Diverticulosis:
Diverticulosis often remains asymptomatic, meaning many people with the condition do not experience any noticeable symptoms. When symptoms do occur, they are typically mild and may include:
- Abdominal Discomfort: Mild cramping or pain, usually in the lower left side of the abdomen.
- Bloating and Gas: Increased gas and a feeling of fullness in the abdomen.
- Changes in Bowel Habits: Occasional changes in bowel movements, such as constipation or diarrhoea.

These symptoms are often intermittent and may be mistaken for other digestive issues, such as irritable bowel syndrome (IBS).

Diverticulitis:
Diverticulitis, on the other hand, involves inflammation or infection of the diverticula and presents more severe and noticeable symptoms. Common symptoms of diverticulitis include:
- Abdominal Pain: Sharp, persistent pain, typically in the lower left quadrant of the abdomen. The pain can be severe and may worsen with movement.

- Fever and Chills: Elevated body temperature and chills indicating infection.
- Nausea and Vomiting: These symptoms often accompany severe abdominal pain.

Changes in Bowel Habits:
Constipation is more common, but diarrhoea can also occur. There may be a noticeable change in the consistency or frequency of bowel movements.
- Tenderness in the Abdomen: The affected area may be tender to touch, and the pain can increase with pressure.
- Bloating and Gas: Similar to diverticulosis, but more pronounced due to inflammation.
- Loss of Appetite: Reduced desire to eat due to pain and discomfort.

Complications:
In severe cases, diverticulitis can lead to complications, such as:
- Abscesses: Pockets of pus that form in the diverticula.
- Perforation: A tear in the colon wall, which can lead to peritonitis (inflammation of the abdominal lining).
- Fistulas: Abnormal connections between the colon and other organs.

- Intestinal Obstruction: Blockage of the bowel.

While diverticulosis is often symptom-free, diverticulitis presents with more severe and acute symptoms that require prompt medical attention. Recognizing these symptoms early can lead to more effective management and treatment, preventing complications and improving patient outcomes.

Managing Symptoms

Effectively managing the symptoms of diverticulosis and diverticulitis is crucial for improving quality of life and preventing complications. Management strategies vary depending on the severity of the symptoms and whether the condition is in the form of diverticulosis or an acute diverticulitis episode.

Diverticulosis Management

Dietary Modifications:
Increase Fibre Intake: A high-fibre diet is essential for managing diverticulosis. Incorporate more fruits, vegetables, whole grains, and legumes into daily meals. Fibre softens stool and promotes regular

bowel movements, reducing pressure on the colon walls.
- Hydration: Drink plenty of water throughout the day to help fibre work effectively and prevent constipation. Aim for at least 8 glasses of water per day.

Lifestyle Changes:
- Regular Exercise: Engage in regular physical activity, such as walking, jogging, or yoga, to stimulate bowel function and reduce the risk of constipation.
- Healthy Weight Management: Maintain a healthy weight to decrease abdominal pressure and reduce the risk of developing more diverticula.

Probiotics:
- Gut Health: Consider incorporating probiotics into your diet through supplements or fermented foods like yogurt, kefir, sauerkraut, and kimchi. Probiotics can help maintain a healthy balance of gut bacteria.

Stress Reduction:
- Stress Management: Practice stress-reducing techniques such as meditation, deep

breathing exercises, or mindfulness to help manage symptoms. Chronic stress can negatively impact gut health and exacerbate symptoms.

Diverticulitis Management

Medical Treatment:
- Antibiotics: For mild to moderate cases of diverticulitis, doctors often prescribe antibiotics to treat infection and reduce inflammation.
- Pain Relief: Over-the-counter pain relievers, such as acetaminophen, can help manage pain. Avoid NSAIDs like ibuprofen, as they can increase the risk of complications.

Dietary Adjustments:
- Clear Liquid Diet: During an acute diverticulitis flare-up, a clear liquid diet may be recommended to allow the colon to heal. This includes broths, clear juices, and water.
- Gradual Reintroduction of Foods: Once symptoms improve, gradually reintroduce low-fibre foods before transitioning back to a high-fibre diet.

Surgery:
- Severe Cases: In cases of severe or recurrent diverticulitis, surgical intervention may be necessary. Surgery typically involves removing the affected portion of the colon to prevent further episodes and complications.

Monitoring and Follow-Up:
- Regular Check-Ups: Regular follow-ups with your healthcare provider are essential to monitor the condition and adjust treatment plans as needed.
- Imaging Tests: In some cases, repeat imaging tests may be necessary to ensure the inflammation or infection has resolved.

Managing the symptoms of diverticulosis and diverticulitis involves a combination of dietary changes, lifestyle modifications, medical treatments, and in some cases, surgical intervention. For diverticulosis, focusing on a high-fibre diet, hydration, regular exercise, and stress management can help prevent complications and improve overall gut health. For diverticulitis, medical treatments, dietary adjustments, and close monitoring are key to managing acute episodes and preventing recurrence. By adopting these strategies, individuals can effectively manage their symptoms and maintain better digestive health.

Importance of early detection

Early detection of diverticulosis and diverticulitis is crucial for effective management, prevention of complications, and improvement of overall health outcomes. Recognizing these conditions in their early stages allows for timely intervention, which can significantly enhance the quality of life for affected individuals.

Preventing Progression:
Early detection of diverticulosis, even when asymptomatic, provides an opportunity to implement dietary and lifestyle changes that can prevent the condition from progressing to diverticulitis. By increasing fibre intake, staying hydrated, and maintaining a healthy lifestyle, individuals can reduce the risk of diverticula becoming inflamed or infected.

Avoiding Complications:
Diverticulitis can lead to serious complications, such as abscesses, perforations, fistulas, and intestinal

obstructions. Detecting and treating diverticulitis early can prevent these potentially life-threatening issues. Prompt medical intervention, including the use of antibiotics and dietary adjustments, can mitigate inflammation and infection before complications arise.

Improving Treatment Outcomes:
Early detection allows for more conservative and less invasive treatment options. For diverticulitis, early intervention often involves antibiotics and dietary modifications, which can be highly effective in managing mild to moderate cases. Late detection, on the other hand, may necessitate more aggressive treatments, such as surgery, which come with higher risks and longer recovery times.

Enhancing Quality of Life:
Living with undiagnosed diverticulosis or unmanaged diverticulitis can lead to chronic pain, discomfort, and a significant decline in quality of life. Early detection and appropriate management can alleviate symptoms, prevent recurrent flare-ups, and enable individuals to maintain a more active and fulfilling lifestyle.

Reducing Healthcare Costs:
Early detection and management can lead to fewer emergency room visits, hospitalizations, and surgical procedures, ultimately reducing healthcare costs for both individuals and the healthcare system. Preventive care and regular monitoring are cost-effective strategies that can minimize the need for more intensive medical interventions.

Promoting Awareness and Education:
Awareness of the importance of early detection can encourage individuals to seek medical advice at the onset of symptoms or during routine health check-ups. Education on the risk factors, symptoms, and preventive measures associated with diverticulosis and diverticulitis can empower people to take proactive steps in maintaining their digestive health.

Early detection of diverticulosis and diverticulitis is vital for preventing progression, avoiding complications, improving treatment outcomes, enhancing quality of life, reducing healthcare costs, and promoting awareness. Recognizing the signs and seeking timely medical attention can make a significant difference in managing these conditions effectively.

Chapter 3

Conventional Treatments

Conventional treatments for diverticulosis and diverticulitis focus on managing symptoms, preventing complications, and promoting overall gut health. These treatments are often the first line of defence and include a combination of dietary changes, medications, and, in severe cases, surgical interventions. Understanding the available conventional treatments helps individuals make informed decisions about their care and work collaboratively with healthcare providers to achieve the best outcomes.

For diverticulosis, the primary goal is to prevent the progression to diverticulitis by addressing underlying factors such as dietary habits and lifestyle choices. Increasing dietary fibre, maintaining adequate hydration, and regular physical activity are cornerstone recommendations. These measures can help reduce the formation of new diverticula and ease symptoms like constipation and abdominal discomfort.

When it comes to **diverticulitis**, treatment becomes more intensive due to the inflammation and infection associated with the condition. Mild to moderate cases of diverticulitis are typically managed with antibiotics, dietary adjustments, and pain relief. More severe cases, especially those involving complications like abscesses or perforations, may require hospitalization and surgical interventions to remove the affected portions of the colon and address any immediate threats to health.

This chapter delves into the specifics of these conventional treatments, providing a comprehensive overview of dietary recommendations, medication regimens, and surgical options. By exploring the full spectrum of conventional treatments, individuals can better understand their condition and actively participate in their treatment plan, ultimately improving their chances for a swift recovery and long-term health maintenance.

Overview of medical treatments

Medical treatments for diverticulosis and diverticulitis are aimed at managing symptoms, preventing complications, and promoting healing. These treatments vary depending on the severity of the condition and the presence of any complications. Here, we provide an overview of the primary medical treatments for both diverticulosis and diverticulitis.

1. Dietary Modifications:
   - High-Fibre Diet: For diverticulosis, increasing dietary fibre intake is crucial. Fibre helps soften stool and promote regular bowel movements, reducing pressure on the colon walls. Foods rich in fibre include fruits, vegetables, whole grains, and legumes.
   - Low-Fibre Diet During Flare-Ups: During an acute diverticulitis episode, a low-fibre or clear liquid diet may be recommended to allow the colon to rest and heal. As symptoms improve, a gradual reintroduction of fibre is essential.

2. Antibiotics:
   - Infection Control: Antibiotics are a primary treatment for mild to moderate cases of diverticulitis. Commonly prescribed antibiotics include metronidazole, ciprofloxacin, and

amoxicillin-coagulant. These medications help reduce infection and inflammation in the diverticula.

3. Pain Management:
   - Over-the-Counter Pain Relievers: Acetaminophen is commonly recommended for managing pain associated with diverticulitis. Nonsteroidal anti-inflammatory drugs (NSAIDs) like ibuprofen should generally be avoided as they can increase the risk of gastrointestinal complications.
   - Prescription Pain Medication: In more severe cases, stronger pain medications may be prescribed under the guidance of a healthcare provider.

4. Hospitalization:
   - Severe Cases: Patients with severe diverticulitis or complications such as abscesses, perforation, or peritonitis may require hospitalization. Intravenous antibiotics, fluids, and close monitoring are provided in a hospital setting.
   - Bowel Rest: In severe cases, bowel rest may be necessary, which involves not eating or

drinking anything by mouth to allow the colon to heal.

5. Surgical Interventions:
    - Elective Surgery: For patients with recurrent or chronic diverticulitis, elective surgery may be considered to remove the affected portion of the colon (colon resection) to prevent future episodes.
    - Emergency Surgery: In cases of severe complications like perforation, abscesses that do not respond to drainage, or significant bleeding, emergency surgery may be required to remove the affected segment of the colon and prevent further complications.

6. Monitoring and Follow-Up:
    - Regular Check-Ups: Regular follow-up appointments with healthcare providers are essential to monitor the condition, assess the effectiveness of treatments, and make necessary adjustments.
    - Colonoscopy: After recovery from an acute episode of diverticulitis, a colonoscopy may be recommended to evaluate the colon and rule out other conditions such as colorectal cancer.

The medical treatments for diverticulosis and diverticulitis range from dietary modifications and antibiotics to pain management and surgical interventions. Each treatment approach is tailored to the severity of the condition and the presence of complications. By understanding these medical treatments, individuals can work closely with their healthcare providers to manage their condition effectively and maintain better digestive health.

Medications and their uses

Medications play a crucial role in managing both diverticulosis and diverticulitis, addressing symptoms, preventing complications, and promoting healing. Here, we provide an overview of the common medications used in treating these conditions and their specific uses.

1. Antibiotics:
Antibiotics are primarily used to treat diverticulitis, particularly when there is evidence of infection or inflammation in the diverticula.
- Metronidazole (Flagyl): This antibiotic is often prescribed for its effectiveness against

anaerobic bacteria that thrive in low-oxygen environments, such as the colon.
- Ciprofloxacin (Cipro): Commonly used in combination with metronidazole, ciprofloxacin targets a broad spectrum of bacteria, including those causing gastrointestinal infections.
- Amoxicillin-Coagulant (Augmentin): This combination antibiotic is effective against a wide range of bacteria and is an alternative to metronidazole and ciprofloxacin.
- Trimethoprim-Sulfamethoxazole (Bactrim): Another alternative used for treating diverticulitis, particularly when patients are allergic to other antibiotics.

2. Pain Relievers:
Pain management is essential in both diverticulosis and diverticulitis to alleviate discomfort and improve quality of life.
- Acetaminophen (Tylenol): Recommended for managing mild to moderate pain associated with diverticulitis. It is preferred over NSAIDs due to its lower risk of causing gastrointestinal complications.
- Opioids: In severe cases, short-term use of opioids like hydrocodone or oxycodone may be necessary to manage intense pain. These

should be used under strict medical supervision due to the risk of dependence and side effects.

3. Antispasmodics:
Antispasmodic medications can help reduce abdominal cramping and discomfort by relaxing the muscles of the gastrointestinal tract.
- Dicyclomine (Bentyl): This medication is used to relieve muscle spasms in the intestines, helping to reduce pain and discomfort.
- Hyoscyamine (Levsin): Another antispasmodic that can help alleviate intestinal cramping and improve bowel function.

4. Anti-inflammatory Drugs:
For managing chronic inflammation associated with diverticulitis, certain anti-inflammatory medications may be prescribed.
- Mesalamine (Asacol, Pentasa): Primarily used for inflammatory bowel diseases, mesalamine can also help reduce inflammation in the colon and prevent recurrent diverticulitis.

5. Stool Softeners and Laxatives:

To prevent constipation and reduce pressure on the colon walls, stool softeners and laxatives may be recommended.
- Docusate Sodium (Colace): A stool softener that makes bowel movements easier and less painful, helping to prevent the formation of new diverticula.
- Polyethylene Glycol (Miralax): An osmotic laxative that draws water into the bowel, making stools softer and easier to pass.

6. Probiotics:
Probiotics can help maintain a healthy balance of gut bacteria, potentially reducing inflammation and promoting overall digestive health.
- Lactobacillus and Bifidobacterium: Common strains found in probiotic supplements and fermented foods like yogurt, kefir, and sauerkraut. They support gut health and may help prevent diverticulitis flare-ups.

7. Anti-diarrheal Medications:
In some cases, diverticulitis may cause diarrhoea, which can be managed with anti-diarrheal medications.
- Loperamide (Imodium): Used to slow down bowel movements and reduce diarrhoea. It

should be used with caution and under medical supervision to avoid complications.

The medications used to treat diverticulosis and diverticulitis include antibiotics, pain relievers, antispasmodics, anti-inflammatory drugs, stool softeners, laxatives, probiotics, and anti-diarrheal medications. Each medication serves a specific purpose, from managing symptoms and reducing inflammation to preventing complications and promoting gut health. Understanding these medications and their uses helps individuals work closely with their healthcare providers to develop an effective treatment plan tailored to their needs.

Surgical options and when they are necessary

Surgical intervention for diverticulosis and diverticulitis is typically reserved for severe cases, complications, or when conservative treatments fail to provide relief. Understanding the surgical options available and when they are necessary can help individuals make informed decisions about their care in collaboration with their healthcare providers.

1. Elective Surgery:
Elective surgery is considered for patients with recurrent or chronic diverticulitis who experience frequent flare-ups or complications that significantly impact their quality of life. The primary elective surgical procedure is a colon resection, also known as a colectomy.
- Partial Colectomy (Colon Resection): This procedure involves removing the affected portion of the colon containing the diverticula and reconnecting the healthy sections of the colon. It is usually performed laparoscopically, which is minimally invasive and associated with shorter recovery times. Elective surgery aims to prevent future episodes of diverticulitis and improve long-term outcomes.

2. Emergency Surgery:
Emergency surgery is necessary in cases of severe complications arising from acute diverticulitis. These complications can be life-threatening and require immediate surgical intervention.
- Abscess Drainage: An abscess, a pocket of pus that forms in the colon, may need to be drained. This can sometimes be done using a

needle guided by imaging (percutaneous drainage), but surgery might be required if the abscess is large or not accessible by less invasive means.
- Hartmann's Procedure: This is often performed in emergency situations where there is a perforation or severe infection. The procedure involves removing the diseased portion of the colon and creating a colostomy, where the end of the colon is brought out through the abdominal wall to allow waste to exit the body into a colostomy bag. The remaining part of the colon is closed off. This procedure can be reversed in a later surgery once the patient has recovered.
- Primary Anastomosis with or without a Protective Stoma: In some cases, the surgeon can remove the diseased section of the colon and immediately reconnect the two ends. Sometimes, a temporary stoma (diverting the bowel through the abdominal wall to allow healing) is also created to protect the reconnected bowel and reduce the risk of complications.

When Surgery is Necessary:

- Recurrent Diverticulitis: Frequent episodes that significantly impact quality of life and do not respond well to medical treatments.
- Complications: Severe complications such as abscesses, fistulas (abnormal connections between the colon and other organs), perforation (a hole in the colon wall), or peritonitis (inflammation of the abdominal lining) necessitate surgical intervention.
- Intestinal Obstruction: Blockages in the colon that prevent the passage of stool and gas, causing severe pain and digestive issues.
- Severe Bleeding: Persistent or severe rectal bleeding that cannot be controlled through other treatments.

Post-Surgical Considerations:

- Recovery and Rehabilitation: Recovery from surgery involves a period of rest and rehabilitation, with gradual reintroduction of normal activities. Follow-up appointments are crucial to monitor healing and address any complications.
- Lifestyle Adjustments: After surgery, patients may need to make dietary and lifestyle

adjustments to support their digestive health and prevent future issues.
- Psychological Support: Dealing with the impact of surgery, especially procedures involving a colostomy, can be challenging. Psychological support and counselling may be beneficial.

Surgical options for diverticulosis and diverticulitis include elective and emergency procedures aimed at removing diseased portions of the colon and addressing severe complications. Surgery is necessary when conservative treatments fail, recurrent episodes occur, or life-threatening complications arise. Understanding these options and their indications helps patients and healthcare providers make informed decisions about the best course of action for managing diverticular disease.

Long-term strategies for maintaining digestive health

Maintaining digestive health is crucial for preventing the recurrence of diverticulitis and managing diverticulosis effectively. Adopting long-term strategies can help keep the digestive system functioning well and reduce the risk of complications. Here are some key strategies to consider:

1. High-Fibre Diet:

Increase Fibre Intake: Consuming a diet rich in fibre is essential for maintaining digestive health. Aim for at least 25-30 grams of fibre daily from sources such as fruits, vegetables, whole grains, and legumes. Fibre helps soften stool, promotes regular bowel movements, and reduces pressure on the colon walls.

Gradual Increase: If you're not used to a high-fibre diet, increase your fibre intake gradually to avoid gas and bloating. This allows your digestive system to adjust.

2. Stay Hydrated:

Drink Plenty of Water: Adequate hydration is vital for digestion and fibre to work effectively. Aim to drink at least 8 glasses (about 2 litres) of water daily. Water helps prevent constipation and keeps the digestive system running smoothly.

3. Regular Exercise:

Physical Activity: Regular exercise stimulates bowel function and helps maintain a healthy weight, both of which are beneficial for digestive health. Aim for at least 30 minutes of moderate exercise, such as walking, swimming, or cycling, most days of the week.

4. Manage Stress:

Stress Reduction Techniques: Chronic stress can negatively impact digestion. Practice stress management techniques such as meditation, yoga, deep breathing exercises, or mindfulness to help reduce stress levels and support digestive health.

5. Probiotics:
Gut Health: Incorporate probiotics into your diet to maintain a healthy balance of gut bacteria. Probiotics can be found in fermented foods like yogurt, kefir, sauerkraut, and kimchi, or taken as supplements. They may help reduce inflammation and promote overall digestive health.

6. Avoid Straining During Bowel Movements:

Healthy Bathroom Habits: Straining can increase pressure on the colon and contribute to the formation of diverticula. Ensure you have enough fibre and water in your diet to make bowel movements easier. If necessary, use a stool softener or a natural laxative as recommended by your healthcare provider.

7. Regular Medical Check-Ups:

Routine Monitoring: Regular check-ups with your healthcare provider are essential to monitor your digestive health and catch any potential issues early. Colonoscopies and other diagnostic tests may be recommended to assess the condition of your colon.

8. Avoid Smoking and Limit Alcohol:

Healthy Lifestyle Choices: Smoking and excessive alcohol consumption can negatively impact digestive health. Avoid smoking and limit alcohol intake to support your overall well-being and reduce the risk of digestive issues.

9. Balanced Diet:

Nutrient-Rich Foods: In addition to fibre, ensure your diet includes a variety of nutrient-rich foods to provide essential vitamins and minerals that support digestive health. Include lean proteins, healthy fats, and a wide range of fruits and vegetables.

10. Listen to Your Body:

Symptom Awareness: Pay attention to your body and recognize any changes in your digestive health. Early detection of symptoms and prompt medical attention can prevent complications and ensure timely treatment.

In summary, maintaining long-term digestive health involves a combination of dietary adjustments, lifestyle changes, and proactive healthcare. By adopting these strategies, individuals with diverticulosis and those recovering from diverticulitis can reduce the risk of recurrence, improve their overall well-being, and enjoy a healthier digestive system.

Chapter 4

Dietary Modifications

Diet plays a crucial role in managing diverticulosis and preventing diverticulitis flare-ups. Making the right dietary choices can significantly improve digestive health, reduce symptoms, and prevent complications. This chapter provides detailed guidelines on dietary modifications that can help maintain a healthy digestive system.

A high-fibre diet is essential for individuals with diverticulosis. Fibre helps soften stool, making it easier to pass and reducing pressure on the colon walls. It also promotes regular bowel movements, preventing constipation, which can exacerbate diverticulosis and lead to diverticulitis. Including a variety of fibre-rich foods such as fruits, vegetables, whole grains, and legumes in your diet can provide the necessary fibre to support digestive health. Fruits like apples, pears, berries, oranges, and bananas, along with vegetables such as broccoli, carrots, spinach, peas, and Brussels sprouts, are excellent sources of dietary fibre. Whole grains like whole wheat bread, brown rice, oatmeal, quinoa, and barley, as well as legumes like beans, lentils, chickpeas, and split peas, can be incorporated into meals to boost fibre intake.

For those not accustomed to a high-fibre diet, it is important to increase fibre intake gradually over several weeks. This gradual increase allows the digestive system to adjust and helps avoid gas and bloating. Adequate hydration is also crucial, as drinking plenty of water helps fibre work effectively and prevents constipation.

During an acute diverticulitis episode, a low-fibre or clear liquid diet may be recommended to allow the colon to rest and heal. Clear liquids such as broths, clear juices, gelation, and water can be consumed initially. Refined grains like white bread, white rice, and plain pasta are easy to digest and can be included in the diet. Cooking and peeling vegetables and fruits can make them easier to digest; cooked carrots, zucchini, and peeled apples are good options. Once symptoms improve, gradually reintroducing fibre into the diet is important, starting with low-fibre foods and slowly incorporating higher-fibre options.

Staying hydrated is essential for digestive health. Adequate hydration helps fibre work effectively and keeps the digestive system running smoothly. Drinking enough water prevents constipation, which can put pressure on the colon and exacerbate diverticulosis. Aim for at least 8 glasses of water per day, adjusting based on activity level, climate, and individual needs. Herbal teas, clear soups, and water-rich fruits and vegetables can also contribute to overall hydration.

Probiotics play a significant role in maintaining a healthy balance of gut bacteria, which can reduce inflammation and improve overall digestive health. Including fermented foods like yogurt, kefir, sauerkraut, kimchi, miso, and tempeh in the diet can provide a good source of probiotics. Probiotic supplements are also available and can be an effective way to ensure adequate intake, especially for those who cannot consume fermented foods.

Identifying and avoiding trigger foods is crucial for managing symptoms. Certain foods may trigger symptoms in some individuals, so keeping a food diary can help identify and eliminate these triggers. Common trigger foods include fatty and fried foods, processed foods, red meat, and foods high in refined sugars. Focusing on a balanced diet with a variety of nutrient-rich foods and avoiding processed and high-fat foods can significantly improve digestive health and reduce symptoms.

Dietary modifications are essential for managing diverticulosis and preventing diverticulitis. A high-fibre diet, proper hydration, the inclusion of probiotics, and avoiding trigger foods can significantly improve digestive health. By making these dietary adjustments, individuals can maintain a healthy digestive system and reduce the risk of complications.

Importance of a high-fibre diet

A high-fibre diet is crucial for managing diverticulosis and preventing diverticulitis flare-ups. Fibre plays several essential roles in maintaining digestive health and overall well-being.

First and foremost, fibre helps soften stool, making it easier to pass and reducing pressure on the colon walls. This is particularly important for individuals with diverticulosis, as increased pressure on the colon can lead to the formation of more diverticula and exacerbate existing ones. Softening the stool and promoting regular bowel movements helps prevent constipation, which is a significant risk factor for diverticulitis.

In addition to its mechanical benefits, fibre supports a healthy balance of gut bacteria. Certain types of fibre, known as prebiotics, serve as food for beneficial gut bacteria, promoting their growth and activity. A healthy gut microbiome is vital for reducing inflammation, enhancing immune function, and preventing infections, all of which are important for individuals with diverticular disease.

Moreover, a high-fibre diet can help manage body weight, which is an important aspect of overall health. High-fibre foods tend to be more filling and can help control appetite, reducing the likelihood of overeating and weight gain. Maintaining a healthy weight reduces the risk of various health conditions, including heart disease, diabetes, and certain types of cancer.

Fibre-rich foods, such as fruits, vegetables, whole grains, and legumes, are also packed with essential vitamins, minerals, and antioxidants. These nutrients support overall health and help protect against chronic diseases. Including a variety of fibre-rich foods in your diet ensures that you receive a broad spectrum of nutrients that are beneficial for your digestive system and overall well-being.

Another important aspect of a high-fibre diet is its ability to regulate blood sugar levels. Soluble fibre, in particular, slows down the absorption of sugar, helping to stabilize blood sugar levels and reduce the risk of type 2 diabetes. For individuals with diverticular disease, maintaining stable blood sugar levels is important, as fluctuations in blood sugar can affect energy levels and overall health.

To reap the benefits of a high-fibre diet, it is important to incorporate a variety of fibre-rich foods into your meals. Fruits like apples, pears, berries, and oranges, as well as vegetables such as broccoli, carrots, spinach, and peas, are excellent sources of dietary fibre. Whole grains like whole wheat bread, brown rice, oatmeal, and quinoa, along with legumes such as beans, lentils, chickpeas, and split peas, can also significantly contribute to your fibre intake.

It is also essential to increase your fibre intake gradually. Sudden increases can cause gas, bloating, and discomfort as your digestive system adjusts. Gradual changes allow your body to adapt and make the transition smoother. Additionally, drinking plenty of water is crucial when increasing fibre intake, as water helps fibre move through the digestive system and prevents constipation.

A high-fibre diet is vital for managing diverticulosis and preventing diverticulitis. It helps soften stool, promotes regular bowel movements, supports a healthy gut microbiome, aids in weight management, provides essential nutrients, regulates blood sugar levels, and reduces the risk of chronic diseases. By incorporating a variety of fibre-rich foods into your diet and increasing fibre intake gradually, you can significantly improve your digestive health and overall well-being.

Foods to avoid and foods to include

Dietary choices play a crucial role in managing diverticulosis and preventing diverticulitis flare-ups. Knowing which foods to avoid and which to include can help maintain a healthy digestive system and reduce the risk of complications.

Foods to Avoid:

1. Processed Foods:

Processed foods are often low in fibre and high in unhealthy fats, sugars, and additives. These foods can contribute to inflammation, poor digestive health, and weight gain, which can exacerbate diverticulosis symptoms. Avoid items such as:
- Fast food
- Packaged snacks (chips, cookies, and crackers)
- Sugary cereals
- Frozen meals and microwave dinners

2. Red Meat and Fatty Foods:

Diets high in red meat and saturated fats are linked to an increased risk of diverticulitis. These foods can be harder to digest and may increase inflammation in the digestive tract. Limit intake of:
- Beef, pork, and lamb
- Bacon and sausages
- High-fat dairy products (whole milk, cream, butter)
- Fried foods

3. Refined Grains:

Refined grains lack the fibre content found in whole grains and can contribute to constipation and

poor digestive health. Avoid products made with white flour, such as:
- White bread and rolls
- White rice
- Regular pasta
- Pastries and baked goods

4. Certain Seeds and Nuts (During Flare-Ups):
While seeds and nuts are generally healthy, some individuals may need to avoid them during an active diverticulitis flare-up, as they can irritate the digestive tract. This includes:
- Popcorn
- Sesame seeds
- Sunflower seeds
- Whole nuts (e.g., almonds, walnuts)

Foods to Include:

1. High-Fibre Foods:
A diet rich in fibre helps soften stool and promotes regular bowel movements, reducing pressure on the colon walls. Include a variety of high-fibre foods such as:
- Fruits: Apples, pears, berries, oranges, bananas

- Vegetables: Broccoli, carrots, spinach, peas, Brussels sprouts
- Whole Grains: Whole wheat bread, brown rice, oatmeal, quinoa, barley
- Legumes: Beans, lentils, chickpeas, split peas

2. Fermented Foods:

Fermented foods contain probiotics that help maintain a healthy balance of gut bacteria, reducing inflammation and promoting overall digestive health. Include foods like:
- Yogurt (with live active cultures)
- Kefir
- Sauerkraut
- Kimchi
- Miso
- Tempeh

3. Lean Proteins:

Opt for lean protein sources that are easier to digest and lower in unhealthy fats. Include options such as:
- Poultry (chicken and turkey)
- Fish and seafood
- Tofu and tempeh
- Legumes and beans

4. Hydration:

Staying hydrated is essential for digestion and helps fibre work effectively. Drink plenty of fluids throughout the day, including:
- Water
- Herbal teas
- Clear broths
- Water-rich fruits and vegetables (cucumbers, watermelon)

5. Healthy Fats:

Incorporate healthy fats that support overall health and reduce inflammation. These include:
- Olive oil
- Avocados
- Nuts and seeds (in moderation)
- Fatty fish (salmon, mackerel)

6. Low-FODMAP Foods (If Necessary):

For some individuals, certain carbohydrates called FODMAPs can exacerbate symptoms. A low-FODMAP diet may help reduce gas, bloating, and discomfort. Foods low in FODMAPs include:
- Bananas, blueberries, and grapes
- Carrots, cucumbers, and zucchini
- Gluten-free grains (rice, quinoa, oats)
- Lactose-free dairy products

Dietary modifications are essential for managing diverticulosis and preventing diverticulitis. Avoid processed foods, red meat, fatty foods, refined grains, and certain seeds and nuts during flare-ups. Instead, focus on a diet rich in high-fibre foods, fermented foods, lean proteins, healthy fats, and low-FODMAP options if necessary. Staying hydrated is also crucial for maintaining digestive health. By making these dietary adjustments, individuals can significantly improve their digestive health and reduce the risk of complications.

Sample meal plans and recipes

Creating a balanced meal plan with a focus on high-fibre foods and other digestive-friendly options can help manage diverticulosis and prevent diverticulitis flare-ups. Below are sample meal plans for three days, along with recipes for some of the dishes.

Day 1
Breakfast:
- Oatmeal with Berries and Almonds

- 1 cup cooked oatmeal
- 1/2 cup mixed berries (blueberries, strawberries, raspberries)
  - 1 tablespoon sliced almonds
  - 1 teaspoon honey (optional)

Mid-Morning Snack:
- Apple Slices with Almond Butter
  - 1 apple, sliced
  - 2 tablespoons almond butter

Lunch:
- Quinoa Salad with Vegetables
  - 1 cup cooked quinoa
  - 1/2 cup cherry tomatoes, halved
  - 1/2 cucumber, diced
  - 1/4 red onion, finely chopped
  - 1/4 cup feta cheese, crumbled
  - 2 tablespoons olive oil
  - 1 tablespoon lemon juice
  - Salt and pepper to taste

Afternoon Snack:
- Greek Yogurt with Honey and Walnuts
  - 1 cup plain Greek yogurt
  - 1 teaspoon honey
  - 1 tablespoon chopped walnuts

Dinner:
- Baked Salmon with Steamed Broccoli and Brown Rice
    - 1 salmon fillet
    - 1 tablespoon olive oil
    - Salt, pepper, and lemon juice to taste
    - 1 cup steamed broccoli
    - 1/2 cup cooked brown rice

Day 2

Breakfast:
- Smoothie with Spinach, Banana, and Chia Seeds
    - 1 cup spinach
    - 1 banana
    - 1/2 cup Greek yogurt
    - 1 tablespoon chia seeds
    - 1 cup almond milk

Mid-Morning Snack:
- Carrot Sticks and Hummus
    - 1 cup carrot sticks
    - 1/4 cup hummus

Lunch:
- Lentil Soup

- 1 cup cooked lentils
- 1/2 cup diced carrots
- 1/2 cup diced celery
- 1/2 cup diced tomatoes
- 4 cups vegetable broth
- 1 tablespoon olive oil
- Salt, pepper, and herbs (thyme, bay leaf) to taste

Afternoon Snack:
- Handful of Mixed Nuts (almonds, walnuts, cashews)

Dinner:
- Grilled Chicken with Roasted Vegetables and Quinoa
    - 1 grilled chicken breast
    - 1 cup roasted vegetables (bell peppers, zucchini, eggplant)
    - 1/2 cup cooked quinoa

Day 3

Breakfast:
- Whole Grain Toast with Avocado and Poached Egg

- 2 slices whole grain toast
- 1/2 avocado, mashed
- 1 poached egg
- Salt, pepper, and red pepper flakes to taste

Mid-Morning Snack:
- Fresh Fruit Salad
    - 1/2 cup diced pineapple
    - 1/2 cup diced mango
    - 1/2 cup diced kiwi

Lunch:
- Chickpea and Spinach Salad
    - 1 cup cooked chickpeas
    - 2 cups spinach leaves
    - 1/2 red bell pepper, sliced
    - 1/4 red onion, thinly sliced
    - 1/4 cup feta cheese, crumbled
    - 2 tablespoons olive oil
    - 1 tablespoon balsamic vinegar
    - Salt and pepper to taste

Afternoon Snack:
- Cottage Cheese with Fresh Berries
    - 1/2 cup cottage cheese
    - 1/2 cup mixed berries (blueberries, raspberries, blackberries)

Dinner:
- Stir-Fried Tofu with Vegetables and Brown Rice
    - 1 cup firm tofu, cubed
    - 1 cup mixed vegetables (broccoli, bell peppers, snap peas)
    - 1 tablespoon soy sauce
    - 1 tablespoon sesame oil
    - 1 garlic clove, minced
    - 1/2 cup cooked brown rice

Recipes

Quinoa Salad with Vegetables

Ingredients:
- 1 cup cooked quinoa
- 1/2 cup cherry tomatoes, halved
- 1/2 cucumber, diced
- 1/4 red onion, finely chopped
- 1/4 cup feta cheese, crumbled
- 2 tablespoons olive oil
- 1 tablespoon lemon juice
- Salt and pepper to taste

Instructions:

1. In a large bowl, combine cooked quinoa, cherry tomatoes, cucumber, red onion, and feta cheese.
2. In a small bowl, whisk together olive oil, lemon juice, salt, and pepper.
3. Pour the dressing over the quinoa mixture and toss to combine.
4. Serve immediately or refrigerate for up to 2 days.

Lentil Soup

Ingredients:
- 1 cup cooked lentils
- 1/2 cup diced carrots
- 1/2 cup diced celery
- 1/2 cup diced tomatoes
- 4 cups vegetable broth
- 1 tablespoon olive oil
- Salt, pepper, and herbs (thyme, bay leaf) to taste

Instructions:
1. In a large pot, heat olive oil over medium heat.
2. Add carrots, celery, and tomatoes, and sauté until tender, about 5-7 minutes.
3. Add cooked lentils and vegetable broth to the pot.
4. Season with salt, pepper, and herbs.
5. Bring the soup to a boil, then reduce heat and simmer for 20-25 minutes.

6. Serve hot with a side of whole grain bread.

Stir-Fried Tofu with Vegetables

Ingredients:
- 1 cup firm tofu, cubed
- 1 cup mixed vegetables (broccoli, bell peppers, snap peas)
- 1 tablespoon soy sauce
- 1 tablespoon sesame oil
- 1 garlic clove, minced
- 1/2 cup cooked brown rice

Instructions:
1. In a large pan or wok, heat sesame oil over medium-high heat.
2. Add garlic and tofu cubes, and stir-fry until tofu is golden brown, about 5-7 minutes.
3. Add mixed vegetables to the pan and continue to stir-fry until tender-crisp, about 5-7 minutes.
4. Add soy sauce and toss to coat the tofu and vegetables evenly.
5. Serve hot over cooked brown rice.

These sample meal plans and recipes focus on incorporating high-fibre foods, lean proteins, healthy fats, and probiotics to support digestive health and manage diverticulosis. By following these guidelines, individuals can enjoy a varied and nutritious diet that helps maintain a healthy digestive system.

Hydration and its role in digestive health

Proper hydration is essential for maintaining overall health, and it plays a particularly crucial role in digestive health. The body relies on water to carry out numerous physiological functions, including digestion and the maintenance of the digestive tract. In the context of managing diverticulosis and preventing diverticulitis, staying adequately hydrated can help mitigate symptoms and support overall digestive function.

Facilitating Digestive Processes:

Water is vital for the entire digestive process, from the moment food enters the mouth until waste is excreted. It aids in the production of saliva, which begins the process of breaking down food and making it easier to swallow. Once food reaches the stomach, water helps dissolve nutrients so they can be absorbed more effectively. In the intestines, water is essential for maintaining the right consistency of stool, making it easier to pass and reducing the risk of constipation.

Preventing Constipation:

Constipation can increase the pressure within the colon, leading to the formation of diverticula and aggravating existing diverticulosis. Adequate hydration helps prevent constipation by softening the stool and promoting regular bowel movements. When the body is well-hydrated, the stool retains more water, which keeps it soft and easy to pass. Conversely, dehydration can lead to hard, dry stools that are difficult to move through the digestive tract, increasing the likelihood of straining and constipation.

Supporting Fibre Function:

A high-fibre diet is essential for managing diverticulosis, but fibre requires water to work effectively. Soluble fibre absorbs water and forms a gel-like substance that helps slow digestion, allowing for better nutrient absorption. Insoluble fibre, on the other hand, adds bulk to the stool and helps move it through the digestive tract more efficiently. Without adequate hydration, fibre can have the opposite effect, leading to hard stools and constipation.

Promoting Gut Health:

Proper hydration is also important for maintaining a healthy balance of gut bacteria. The gut microbiome, which consists of trillions of microorganisms, plays a significant role in digestive health, immune function, and overall well-being. Water helps maintain the environment in which these beneficial bacteria thrive. A healthy, hydrated gut supports the growth and function of these microorganisms, aiding in digestion and reducing inflammation.

Detoxification:

Water assists in the elimination of waste products from the body through urine and sweat. Staying hydrated ensures that the kidneys can effectively filter out toxins and waste products from the blood. Efficient waste removal is important for overall health and can prevent the build-up of harmful substances that may negatively affect the digestive system.

Hydration Tips:

1. Drink Plenty of Water: Aim for at least 8 glasses of water a day, adjusting for factors such as activity level, climate, and individual needs.
2. Monitor Your Hydration: Check the colon of your urine as a simple indicator of hydration. Pale yellow urine typically signifies adequate hydration, while dark yellow or amber can indicate dehydration.
3. Incorporate Water-Rich Foods:
Include fruits and vegetables with high water content in your diet, such as cucumbers, watermelon, oranges, and strawberries.
4. Limit Diuretics: Be mindful of consuming beverages that have a diuretic effect, such as coffee, tea, and alcohol, as they can increase water loss.
5. Set Reminders: Use alarms or apps to remind yourself to drink water throughout the day, especially if you have a busy schedule.

Hydration is a fundamental aspect of digestive health. It facilitates the entire digestive process, prevents constipation, supports the function of dietary fibre, promotes a healthy gut microbiome, and aids in detoxification. By prioritizing adequate water intake and incorporating water-rich foods into your diet, you can support your digestive system and effectively manage diverticulosis.

Chapter 5

Natural Remedies and Supplements

Natural remedies and supplements can play a crucial role in managing diverticulosis and preventing diverticulitis flare-ups. While conventional treatments and dietary modifications are essential, integrating natural approaches offers a holistic way to support digestive health and overall well-being. This chapter delves into various natural strategies that can complement traditional medical care, providing additional relief and promoting a healthier digestive system.

Probiotics and prebiotics are fundamental in maintaining a balanced gut microbiome, which is essential for digestive health. Probiotics, found in fermented foods like yogurt and kefir, introduce beneficial bacteria into the gut, while prebiotics, present in foods such as garlic and onions, feed these good bacteria, fostering a healthy environment. Together, they can help reduce inflammation and enhance immune function.

Herbal remedies such as peppermint, ginger, and turmeric have anti-inflammatory and soothing properties that can alleviate digestive discomfort. These herbs can be consumed in various forms, including teas, capsules, and fresh additions to meals. They offer natural ways to reduce symptoms like bloating, gas, and nausea.

Fibre supplements can also be beneficial, especially for those struggling to meet their fibre needs through diet alone. Supplements like psyllium husk and inulin help maintain regular bowel movements and prevent constipation, a key factor in managing diverticulosis.

Essential nutrients like omega-3 fatty acids and vitamin D contribute to reducing inflammation and supporting overall health. Omega-3s, found in fish oil and flaxseeds, and vitamin D, obtained through sunlight and supplements, are crucial for a balanced diet and healthy digestion.

Mind-body practices such as yoga, meditation, and regular physical activity can reduce stress, which is closely linked to digestive health. Staying well-hydrated also plays a vital role, ensuring that fibre can work effectively in the digestive tract.

By integrating these natural remedies and supplements into daily routines, individuals with diverticular disease can enhance their digestive health, reduce the frequency of flare-ups, and improve their overall quality of life.

Herbal remedies and their benefits

Herbal remedies have been used for centuries to treat various ailments, including digestive disorders. For individuals with diverticulosis and diverticulitis, certain herbs can offer significant relief by reducing inflammation, soothing the digestive tract, and promoting overall digestive health. Here, we explore some of the most effective herbal remedies and their benefits.

Peppermint

Peppermint is well-known for its soothing effects on the digestive system. It contains menthol, which has antispasmodic properties that help relax the muscles of the gastrointestinal tract, reducing symptoms such as bloating, gas, and cramping. Peppermint tea is a popular way to consume this herb, but peppermint oil capsules, especially those that are enteric-coated, can provide targeted relief for symptoms of irritable bowel syndrome (IBS), which often overlaps with diverticular disease.

Ginger

Ginger is another powerful herb with numerous benefits for digestive health. It has anti-inflammatory and antioxidant properties, which can help reduce inflammation in the gut. Ginger is particularly effective in alleviating nausea, vomiting, and indigestion. Fresh ginger can be added to meals or brewed into tea, and ginger supplements are also widely available. Consuming ginger regularly can support digestive motility and reduce discomfort associated with digestive disorders.

Turmeric

Turmeric contains curcumin, a compound with strong anti-inflammatory and antioxidant properties. Curcumin can help reduce inflammation in the digestive tract, which is beneficial for individuals with diverticulosis and diverticulitis. Turmeric can be incorporated into the diet as a spice in cooking, or it can be taken as a supplement. When using supplements, it's often recommended to choose those with added black pepper extract (pipevine) to enhance curcuma absorption.

Chamomile

Chamomile is known for its calming effects, but it also offers digestive benefits. It has anti-inflammatory, antispasmodic, and carminative properties, making it effective in relieving gas, bloating, and cramps. Chamomile tea is a gentle and soothing way to consume this herb, providing relief from digestive discomfort and promoting relaxation, which can be particularly beneficial during episodes of digestive distress.

Fennel

Fennel seeds have been traditionally used to aid digestion and alleviate symptoms such as bloating, gas, and abdominal cramps. They contain compounds like anethole, which has antispasmodic and anti-inflammatory effects. Chewing fennel seeds after meals or drinking fennel tea can help stimulate digestion and reduce digestive discomfort.

Slippery Elm

Slippery elm is a mucilaginous herb that forms a gel-like substance when mixed with water. This gel can coat and soothe the lining of the digestive tract, reducing irritation and inflammation. Slippery elm is particularly helpful for individuals with inflammatory bowel conditions, as it can help protect the mucous membranes of the gut. It is available in powder, capsule, and lozenge forms, and can be taken with water or added to smoothies.

Marshmallow Root

Similar to slippery elm, marshmallow root has mucilaginous properties that can soothe and protect the digestive tract. It helps reduce inflammation and irritation, making it beneficial for individuals with diverticular disease. Marshmallow root can be consumed as a tea or taken in supplement form to support digestive health.

Liquorice Root

Liquorice root, particularly deglycyrrhizinated licorice (DGL), has anti-inflammatory and soothing properties that can benefit the digestive system. It helps protect the mucous membranes and reduce inflammation in the gut. DGL is often used to treat conditions such as gastritis and peptic ulcers, and it can also be beneficial for individuals with diverticulosis. It is available in chewable tablets and can be taken before meals to support digestive health.

Aloe Vera

Aloe Vera juice is known for its soothing and anti-inflammatory properties. It can help reduce inflammation in the digestive tract and promote healing. Aloe Vera juice is gentle on the stomach and can be consumed daily to support overall digestive health. It's important to choose a high-quality, pure aloe Vera juice without added sugars or artificial ingredients.

Herbal remedies offer a natural and effective way to support digestive health and manage symptoms of diverticulosis and diverticulitis. Herbs like peppermint, ginger, turmeric, chamomile, fennel, slippery elm, marshmallow root, licorice root, and aloe Vera have various properties that can reduce inflammation, soothe the digestive tract, and promote overall well-being. Incorporating these herbs into your daily routine, whether through teas, supplements, or fresh additions to meals, can provide significant relief and enhance your digestive health. As with any natural remedy, it's important to consult with a healthcare provider before starting any new herbal supplement to ensure it's appropriate for your individual needs.

Probiotics and prebiotics

Probiotics and prebiotics play a crucial role in maintaining gut health, which is essential for managing diverticulosis and preventing diverticulitis flare-ups. Understanding their functions, benefits, and sources can help individuals effectively incorporate them into their daily routines for better digestive health.

Probiotics: The Beneficial Bacteria

Probiotics are live microorganisms, often referred to as "good" or "friendly" bacteria, that provide health benefits when consumed in adequate amounts. They help maintain a healthy balance of gut microbiota, which is essential for optimal digestive function, immune support, and overall health. Probiotics can be found in certain foods and dietary supplements.

Benefits of Probiotics:

1. Restoring Gut Balance: Probiotics help replenish beneficial bacteria in the gut, especially after disruptions caused by antibiotics, illness, or poor diet. This balance is crucial for preventing overgrowth of harmful bacteria and promoting a healthy digestive environment.

2. Enhancing Digestion: Probiotics aid in the breakdown and absorption of nutrients, improving overall digestive efficiency. They can help alleviate symptoms like bloating, gas, and constipation by promoting regular bowel movements.

3. Reducing Inflammation: Certain probiotic strains have anti-inflammatory properties that can help reduce inflammation in the gut, which is beneficial for individuals with diverticulosis and other inflammatory bowel conditions.

4. Supporting Immune Function: A significant portion of the immune system is located in the gut.

Probiotics can enhance immune responses, helping the body defend against pathogens and reducing the risk of infections.

Sources of Probiotics:

- Yogurt: A well-known source of probiotics, yogurt contains live cultures of beneficial bacteria such as Lactobacillus and Bifidobacterium. Look for labels that state "live and active cultures" to ensure probiotic content.
- Kefir: A fermented dairy product similar to yogurt, kefir contains a diverse range of probiotic strains. It can be consumed as a drink or added to smoothies.

Sauerkraut: Fermented cabbage, sauerkraut is rich in probiotics and fibber. It's important to choose unpasteurized sauerkraut to retain the live bacteria.

- Kimchi: A traditional Korean dish made from fermented vegetables, kimchi offers a variety of probiotics and can be a flavourful addition to meals.
- Miso: A fermented soybean paste, miso is used in soups and sauces. It contains probiotics that support gut health.

Probiotic Supplements: Available in various forms such as capsules, tablets, and powders, probiotic supplements can provide a concentrated dose of beneficial bacteria. It's important to choose high-quality supplements with multiple strains for optimal benefits.

Prebiotics: The Food for Probiotics

Prebiotics are non-digestible fibres that act as food for probiotics, promoting the growth and activity of beneficial bacteria in the gut. Unlike probiotics, which are live microorganisms, prebiotics are found in various plant-based foods.

Benefits of Prebiotics:

1. Feeding Beneficial Bacteria: Prebiotics serve as a food source for probiotics, helping them thrive and multiply in the gut. This symbiotic relationship enhances the overall balance of the gut microbiota.

2. Improving Digestive Health: By promoting the growth of beneficial bacteria, prebiotics help maintain a healthy gut environment. They can improve bowel regularity and reduce symptoms such as constipation and bloating.

3. Enhancing Mineral Absorption: Prebiotics can improve the absorption of essential minerals such as calcium and magnesium, supporting overall health and bone strength.

4. Supporting Immune Function: A healthy gut microbiome, supported by prebiotics, contributes to a stronger immune system and better overall health.

Sources of Prebiotics:

- Garlic: Contains inulin, a type of prebiotic fibre that supports the growth of beneficial bacteria.
- Onions: Rich in prebiotic fibres like inulin and fructooligosaccharides (FOS), onions promote gut health.
- Leeks: Another excellent source of inulin, leeks can be added to soups, stews, and salads.
- Asparagus: High in prebiotic fibres, asparagus supports the growth of beneficial bacteria.
- Bananas: Especially when slightly green, bananas contain prebiotic fibres that feed probiotics.

- Chicory Root: A rich source of inulin, chicory root is often used as a coffee substitute and can be added to foods and beverages.
- Jerusalem Artichokes: Also known as sun chokes, these tubers are high in inulin and can be roasted or added to salads.
- Whole Grains: Foods like oats, barley, and wheat contain prebiotic fibres that support gut health.

Incorporating probiotics and prebiotics into your diet is essential for maintaining a healthy gut microbiome, which is crucial for managing diverticulosis and preventing diverticulitis flare-ups. Probiotics provide beneficial bacteria that enhance digestion, reduce inflammation, and support immune function, while prebiotics feed these beneficial bacteria, promoting their growth and activity. By consuming a variety of probiotic-rich foods and prebiotic fibres, or using high-quality supplements, you can create a balanced and supportive environment for your gut, leading to improved digestive health and overall well-being. Always consult with a healthcare provider before starting any new supplement regimen to ensure it aligns with your individual health needs.

Vitamins and minerals essential for gut health

Vitamins and minerals play a crucial role in maintaining gut health and overall well-being. A balanced intake of these essential nutrients supports digestive function, reduces inflammation, and promotes a healthy gut microbiome. This section explores the key vitamins and minerals that are particularly beneficial for gut health, their roles, sources, and how they contribute to optimal digestive function.

1. Vitamin D

Role in Gut Health:
Vitamin D is vital for maintaining a healthy gut microbiome and supporting the immune system. It helps regulate the expression of antimicrobial peptides, which are crucial for defending against pathogens in the gut. Adequate vitamin D levels can also reduce inflammation and support the integrity of the gut barrier, preventing conditions like leaky gut syndrome.

Sources:

- Sunlight: The body synthesizes vitamin D in response to sunlight exposure. Aim for at least 10-30 minutes of sun exposure several times a week, depending on skin type and geographic location.
- Fatty Fish: Salmon, mackerel, and sardines are excellent sources of vitamin D.
- Fortified Foods: Many dairy products, orange juice, and cereals are fortified with vitamin D.
- Supplements: Vitamin D3 supplements are a common choice, especially in areas with limited sunlight.

2. Vitamin A

Role in Gut Health:
Vitamin A is crucial for maintaining the health of the intestinal mucosa, which is the lining of the gut. It supports the regeneration of epithelial cells and helps prevent infections by maintaining the integrity of the gut barrier. Vitamin A also plays a role in immune function and reducing inflammation.

Sources:
- Carrots and Sweet Potatoes: Rich in beta-carotene, which the body converts into vitamin A.

- Leafy Greens: Spinach and kale are good sources of vitamin A.
- Animal Liver: Liver from beef, chicken, and other animals is high in preformed vitamin A (retinol).
- Fortified Foods: Some dairy products and cereals are fortified with vitamin A.

3. Vitamin C

Role in Gut Health:
Vitamin C is a powerful antioxidant that helps protect the gut lining from oxidative stress and inflammation. It also supports the immune system and enhances the absorption of non-heme iron from plant-based foods, which is important for maintaining overall health and energy levels.

Sources:
- Citrus Fruits: Oranges, grapefruits, and lemons are high in vitamin C.
- Berries: Strawberries, blueberries, and raspberries are excellent sources.
- Bell Peppers: Red and green bell peppers contain significant amounts of vitamin C.

- Broccoli and Brussels Sprouts: These vegetables are also good sources of vitamin C.

4. Vitamin B12

Role in Gut Health:
Vitamin B12 is essential for nerve function and the production of red blood cells. It also supports the health of the gut lining and aids in the digestion and absorption of nutrients. Deficiency in vitamin B12 can lead to gastrointestinal symptoms such as constipation and loss of appetite.

Sources:
- Animal Products: Meat, poultry, fish, eggs, and dairy products are rich in vitamin B12.
- Fortified Foods: Some plant-based milks and cereals are fortified with vitamin B12.
- Supplements: Vitamin B12 supplements are available in various forms, including oral tablets and sublingual (under-the-tongue) forms.

5. Magnesium

Role in Gut Health:

Magnesium plays a role in muscle function, including the muscles of the digestive tract. It helps regulate bowel movements by relaxing the intestinal muscles and promoting normal peristalsis (the wave-like contractions that move food through the digestive tract). Magnesium also helps manage stress, which can impact gut health.

Sources:
- Nuts and Seeds: Almonds, cashews, and pumpkin seeds are high in magnesium.
- Leafy Greens: Spinach and Swiss chard provide substantial amounts of magnesium.
- Whole Grains: Brown rice, quinoa, and whole wheat are good sources.
- Legumes: Beans, lentils, and chickpeas are rich in magnesium.

6. Zinc

Role in Gut Health:
Zinc is crucial for maintaining the health of the gut lining and supporting immune function. It aids in the repair of intestinal cells and helps regulate inflammation. Adequate zinc levels are important for preventing gut permeability issues and supporting overall digestive health.

Sources:
- Meat: Beef, pork, and lamb are rich sources of zinc.
- Shellfish: Oysters, crab, and lobster provide high amounts of zinc.
- Nuts and Seeds: Pumpkin seeds, cashews, and hemp seeds are good sources.
- Legumes: Chickpeas, lentils, and beans contain zinc.

7. Iron

Role in Gut Health:
Iron is essential for the production of haemoglobin, which carries oxygen to cells throughout the body. It also supports the health of the gut lining and aids in the absorption of other nutrients. Iron deficiency can lead to fatigue and digestive issues, including changes in bowel movements.

Sources:
- Red Meat: Beef and lamb are rich in heme iron, which is easily absorbed by the body.
- Poultry and Fish: Chicken and fish also provide heme iron.

- Plant-Based Sources: Spinach, lentils, and fortified cereals contain non-heme iron, which is less readily absorbed but can be enhanced by consuming vitamin C-rich foods.

Vitamins and minerals are vital for maintaining optimal gut health and overall well-being. Essential nutrients like vitamin D, vitamin A, vitamin C, vitamin B12, magnesium, zinc, and iron each play unique roles in supporting digestive function, reducing inflammation, and promoting a healthy gut microbiome. Incorporating a diverse range of nutrient-rich foods into your diet, or using supplements when necessary, can help ensure you meet your daily requirements and support a healthy digestive system. Always consult with a healthcare provider before starting any new supplement regimen to address individual health needs and avoid potential interactions.

Chapter 6

Lifestyle Changes for Better Digestive Health

Lifestyle changes play a crucial role in maintaining and improving digestive health, especially for individuals with diverticulosis and diverticulitis. Embracing a holistic approach that integrates healthy habits can significantly reduce the risk of flare-ups, alleviate symptoms, and promote overall well-being. This chapter explores how various lifestyle modifications can create a supportive environment for optimal digestive function.

Firstly, physical activity is essential for digestive health. Regular exercise stimulates the muscles in the digestive tract, promoting regular bowel movements and preventing constipation. Additionally, physical activity helps maintain a healthy weight, which is important for reducing pressure on the intestines and preventing the formation of diverticula.

Managing stress is another critical factor. Chronic stress can negatively impact the gut, leading to issues such as increased gut permeability, inflammation, and altered gut motility. Incorporating stress-reduction techniques such as mindfulness, meditation, yoga, and deep breathing exercises can help manage stress levels and support a healthier digestive system.

Adequate sleep is also vital for digestive health. Poor sleep can disrupt the balance of gut bacteria and impair the digestive process. Establishing a regular sleep routine and ensuring sufficient rest each night can contribute to better digestive function and overall health.

Hydration is key to maintaining digestive health. Drinking enough water helps dissolve soluble fibre and fats, making it easier for the digestive system to process food. It also aids in preventing constipation by keeping the stool soft and easier to pass.

Lastly, avoiding smoking and excessive alcohol consumption is crucial. Both habits can harm the digestive tract, increase inflammation, and exacerbate symptoms of diverticulosis and diverticulitis. By making these lifestyle changes, individuals can create a healthier environment for their digestive system, leading to improved gut health and overall quality of life.

Exercise and physical activity

Regular exercise and physical activity are fundamental components of maintaining and improving digestive health, particularly for individuals with diverticulosis and diverticulitis. Engaging in consistent physical activity not only supports overall health but also directly benefits the digestive system in several ways. Understanding the relationship between exercise and digestive health can empower individuals to incorporate effective physical activity routines into their daily lives.

One of the primary benefits of regular exercise is the stimulation of the digestive tract. Physical activity increases blood flow to the muscles of the digestive system, which enhances the efficiency of intestinal contractions, known as peristalsis. This process helps move food through the digestive tract more smoothly and prevents issues such as constipation and bloating. Improved peristalsis can reduce the risk of developing diverticula (small pouches that can form in the walls of the colon) and can help manage symptoms in those already diagnosed with diverticulosis.

Moreover, regular physical activity helps maintain a healthy weight, which is crucial for digestive health. Excess body weight, especially around the abdomen, can put pressure on the intestines and increase the risk of diverticular disease. By engaging in regular exercise, individuals can manage their weight more effectively, reducing the strain on their digestive organs and promoting a healthier gut environment.

Exercise also plays a significant role in reducing stress, which has a profound impact on digestive health. Chronic stress can lead to disruptions in the gut-brain axis, resulting in gastrointestinal issues such as irritable bowel syndrome (IBS), increased gut permeability, and inflammation. Physical activity is a natural stress reliever, as it promotes the release of endorphins—chemicals in the brain that act as natural painkillers and mood elevators. Activities such as yoga, tai chi, and moderate aerobic exercise like walking, swimming, or cycling can be particularly effective in reducing stress levels and supporting a healthier digestive system.

In addition to these benefits, regular exercise can help regulate bowel movements. For individuals with diverticulosis, maintaining regular bowel movements is essential to avoid constipation and the formation of hard stools, which can irritate the diverticula and lead to diverticulitis. Aerobic exercises, such as jogging, brisk walking, and dancing, help stimulate the natural contractions of intestinal muscles, promoting regular and healthy bowel movements.

Furthermore, engaging in physical activity can enhance the diversity and health of the gut microbiome. Studies have shown that regular exercise can increase the abundance of beneficial bacteria in the gut, which play a crucial role in digestion, immune function, and overall health. A healthy and diverse gut microbiome can help reduce inflammation and improve the body's ability to fight off infections, including those that might affect the digestive tract.

To maximize the benefits of exercise for digestive health, it is important to incorporate a variety of activities into one's routine. This can include a mix of aerobic exercises, strength training, and flexibility exercises. Aiming for at least 150 minutes of moderate aerobic activity or 75 minutes of vigorous activity per week, combined with muscle-strengthening activities on two or more days a week, can provide substantial health benefits.

Regular exercise and physical activity are vital for maintaining and improving digestive health. By promoting efficient digestion, reducing stress, maintaining a healthy weight, regulating bowel movements, and supporting a diverse gut microbiome, exercise offers numerous benefits that can help manage and prevent diverticulosis and diverticulitis. Incorporating regular physical activity into daily life can lead to a healthier, more balanced digestive system and overall well-being.

Physical activities that is helpful

1. Walking:
   - Easy and accessible for most people
   - Promotes gentle movement of food through the digestive tract

2. Jogging or Running:

- Increases overall fitness
- Stimulates intestinal contractions

3. Swimming:
   - Low-impact and easy on the joints
   - Full-body workout that enhances digestion

4. Cycling:
   - Good cardiovascular exercise
   - Helps regulate bowel movements

5. Yoga:
   - Combines physical activity with relaxation techniques
   - Specific poses can aid digestion and reduce stress

6. Tai Chi:
   - Gentle movements and breath control
   - Improves circulation and reduces stress

7. Pilates:
   - Strengthens core muscles
   - Enhances overall digestive function

8. Strength Training:

- Builds muscle mass and increases metabolism
- Supports overall physical health and digestive efficiency

9. Dancing:
    - Fun and engaging way to stay active
    - Increases heart rate and stimulates digestion

10. Hiking:
    - Combines cardiovascular exercise with the benefits of being outdoors
    - Promotes physical fitness and mental well-being

Regular engagement in these activities can support digestive health, reduce the risk of complications related to diverticulosis, and enhance overall well-being.

Stress management techniques

Managing stress is crucial for maintaining digestive health, especially for individuals with diverticulosis and diverticulitis. Chronic stress can negatively impact the gut, leading to symptoms such as increased gut permeability, inflammation, and altered gut motility. Implementing effective stress management techniques can significantly improve digestive health and overall well-being.

1. Mindfulness and Meditation:
Mindfulness and meditation are powerful techniques for reducing stress and promoting relaxation. Mindfulness involves focusing on the present moment and accepting it without judgment. This practice can help individuals become more aware of their stress triggers and responses, allowing them to manage stress more effectively. Meditation, particularly mindfulness meditation, involves sitting quietly, focusing on the breath, and observing thoughts without getting caught up in them. Regular meditation practice can lower stress hormones, reduce inflammation, and improve overall mental and physical health.

2. Deep Breathing Exercises:
Deep breathing exercises can help activate the body's relaxation response, reducing stress and promoting a sense of calm. Techniques such as diaphragmatic breathing, where you breathe deeply into the abdomen rather than shallowly into the chest, can slow the heart rate, lower blood

pressure, and relax the muscles. Practicing deep breathing for a few minutes each day or during stressful moments can be an effective way to manage stress.

3. Physical Activity:
Regular physical activity is a natural stress reliever. Exercise promotes the release of endorphins, chemicals in the brain that act as natural painkillers and mood elevators. Activities such as walking, jogging, swimming, and yoga can reduce stress levels, improve mood, and enhance overall well-being. Even a short daily walk can have significant stress-reducing benefits.

4. Yoga and Tai Chi:
Yoga and Tai Chi combine physical movement with mindfulness and deep breathing, making them excellent practices for stress management. Yoga involves a series of postures and stretches that improve flexibility, strength, and relaxation. Tai Chi, a form of martial arts, focuses on slow, deliberate movements and breath control. Both practices can reduce stress, improve mental clarity, and promote a sense of inner peace.

5. Progressive Muscle Relaxation (PMR):

Progressive Muscle Relaxation involves tensing and then slowly relaxing different muscle groups in the body. This technique can help individuals become more aware of physical tension associated with stress and learn how to release it. Practicing PMR regularly can lead to reduced overall stress levels and improved relaxation.

6. Engaging in Hobbies:
Engaging in hobbies and activities that bring joy and relaxation can be an effective way to manage stress. Whether it's reading, gardening, painting, or listening to music, taking time for enjoyable activities can provide a mental break from stressors and improve overall mood.

7. Social Support:
Building and maintaining strong social connections is vital for managing stress. Talking to friends, family, or a therapist about stressors can provide emotional support, offer different perspectives, and help reduce feelings of isolation. Social interactions can also stimulate the release of oxytocin, a hormone that promotes feelings of bonding and relaxation.

Incorporating these stress management techniques into daily life can lead to a significant reduction in stress levels, promoting better digestive health and overall well-being. By actively managing stress, individuals with diverticulosis and diverticulitis can create a more supportive environment for their digestive systems, reducing the risk of flare-ups and improving quality of life.

How to prevent diverticulosis from progressing to diverticulitis

Preventing diverticulosis from progressing to diverticulitis involves adopting a proactive approach to maintaining gut health and managing risk factors. Diverticulosis, characterized by the presence of small pouches (diverticula) in the colon, can escalate to diverticulitis if these pouches become inflamed or infected. Here are key strategies to prevent this progression.

1. Dietary Modifications:
A high-fibre diet is crucial for preventing diverticulitis. Fibre helps soften and add bulk to stool, promoting regular bowel movements and

reducing pressure on the colon. Incorporate plenty of fruits, vegetables, whole grains, and legumes into your diet. These foods not only provide essential fibre but also deliver important vitamins and minerals that support overall digestive health. Aim for a daily fibre intake of 25-30 grams. Gradually increase fibre intake to avoid bloating and gas, and ensure adequate hydration to help fibre move smoothly through the digestive system.

2. Stay Hydrated:
Drinking plenty of water is essential for maintaining healthy digestion. Adequate hydration helps soften stool and prevents constipation, reducing the risk of diverticula becoming inflamed. Aim for at least eight 8-ounce glasses of water a day, and adjust based on activity level and climate.

3. Regular Physical Activity:
Exercise promotes healthy digestion by stimulating intestinal contractions and reducing the time it takes for food to move through the colon. Regular physical activity can help prevent constipation and reduce pressure on the colon. Aim for at least 150 minutes of moderate-intensity exercise, such as walking, swimming, or cycling, each week.

4. Avoid Straining During Bowel Movements:
Straining can increase pressure in the colon and contribute to the formation of diverticula or aggravate existing ones. To avoid straining, ensure you maintain a diet high in fibre, stay hydrated, and respond promptly to the urge to have a bowel movement.

5. Limit Red Meat and High-Fat Foods:
A diet high in red meat and fatty foods has been associated with an increased risk of diverticulitis. Reducing intake of these foods and opting for lean proteins, such as poultry and fish, and healthy fats, like those found in nuts and avocados, can support gut health.

6. Manage Stress:
Chronic stress can negatively impact digestion and gut health. Implementing stress management techniques, such as mindfulness, meditation, and yoga, can help maintain a healthy digestive system.

By incorporating these lifestyle changes and dietary adjustments, individuals with diverticulosis can significantly reduce the risk of progression to diverticulitis, supporting long-term digestive health and overall well-being.

Regular medical check-ups and monitoring

Regular medical check-ups and monitoring are essential for individuals
with diverticulosis to prevent the condition from progressing to diverticulitis. Routine check-ups allow healthcare providers to keep track of any changes in the digestive system, identify early signs of complications, and provide timely interventions.

During medical appointments, doctors can perform physical examinations and recommend diagnostic tests, such as colonoscopies, to monitor the condition of the colon. These tests can detect any new or worsening diverticula, inflammation, or other abnormalities that might indicate an increased risk of diverticulitis.

Healthcare providers can also offer personalized advice on managing diverticulosis through diet, lifestyle changes, and medications if necessary. They can assess the effectiveness of current management strategies and make adjustments based on the patient's progress and any new symptoms.

Furthermore, regular monitoring ensures that any flare-ups or signs of infection are promptly addressed, reducing the risk of severe complications. Early detection and intervention can significantly improve outcomes and maintain the patient's quality of life.

By prioritizing regular medical check-ups and monitoring, individuals with diverticulosis can stay proactive in managing their condition and preventing its progression to diverticulitis.

Chapter 7

Holistic Approaches to Healing

In addressing diverticulosis and diverticulitis, a holistic approach to healing considers the interconnectedness of the body, mind, and spirit. This chapter explores the various holistic strategies that can complement conventional medical treatments and support overall well-being. By integrating practices such as stress management, dietary modifications, physical activity, and alternative therapies, individuals can create a comprehensive plan to enhance digestive health and prevent flare-ups.

Holistic healing emphasizes the importance of treating the whole person rather than just the symptoms of a disease. It involves recognizing the impact of lifestyle, emotional health, and environmental factors on physical well-being. For those managing diverticulosis and diverticulitis, adopting a holistic approach can lead to more sustainable and effective outcomes.

This chapter will delve into several key areas, including the role of nutrition, the benefits of stress reduction techniques, the impact of regular physical activity, and the use of natural remedies and supplements. We will also discuss the importance of mental and emotional health in the healing process and how practices such as mindfulness, meditation, and alternative therapies can support digestive health.

By embracing a holistic approach, individuals can take proactive steps to manage their condition, reduce symptoms, and improve their quality of life. This comprehensive strategy not only addresses the immediate needs of the digestive system but also fosters long-term health and resilience.

Integrative medicine and its role in treatment

Integrative medicine combines conventional medical treatments with complementary and alternative therapies to address the whole person, focusing on physical, emotional, mental, and spiritual health. This approach recognizes that combining different therapeutic modalities can offer more comprehensive and effective care for conditions like diverticulosis and diverticulitis.

1. Combining Conventional and Complementary Treatments:
Integrative medicine does not replace conventional treatments but rather complements them. For example, while antibiotics and surgery might be necessary for acute diverticulitis, integrating dietary changes, stress management techniques, and herbal supplements can enhance recovery and prevent recurrence. This synergistic approach can help reduce the severity and frequency of flare-ups by addressing the root causes and contributing factors.

2. Personalized Care:
One of the hallmarks of integrative medicine is its emphasis on personalized care. Each individual's condition and lifestyle are unique, and integrative medicine practitioners tailor treatment plans to fit the specific needs of the patient. This might include personalized nutrition plans, exercise routines, stress reduction techniques, and the use of specific supplements or herbal remedies that are most appropriate for the individual's symptoms and overall health.

3. Nutrition and Dietary Support:
A significant component of integrative medicine for managing diverticulosis and diverticulitis is nutrition. Integrative practitioners often work with patients to develop high-fibre diets that include fruits, vegetables, whole grains, and legumes, which are essential for preventing constipation and maintaining colon health. They may also recommend eliminating foods that irritate the gut, such as processed foods, red meat, and high-fat items, and replacing them with anti-inflammatory and gut-healing foods.

4. Stress Management:
Stress is a major factor that can exacerbate digestive disorders. Integrative medicine incorporates stress management techniques such as mindfulness, meditation, yoga, and deep breathing exercises into treatment plans. These practices not only help reduce stress but also improve overall mental and emotional well-being, which in turn supports digestive health.

5. Natural Remedies and Supplements:
Integrative medicine often includes the use of natural remedies and supplements to support

digestive health. For example, probiotics and prebiotics can help maintain a healthy gut microbiome, while herbal remedies like peppermint oil and ginger can soothe the digestive tract. Vitamins and minerals, such as vitamin D and magnesium, may also be recommended to support overall health and digestion.

6. Mind-Body Therapies:
Mind-body therapies, such as acupuncture, massage therapy, and biofeedback, are commonly used in integrative medicine. These therapies can help alleviate pain, reduce stress, and improve overall well-being. Acupuncture, for instance, has been shown to reduce inflammation and promote healing in the digestive tract.

7. Holistic Lifestyle Changes:
Integrative medicine encourages holistic lifestyle changes that promote long-term health. This includes regular physical activity, adequate sleep, proper hydration, and avoiding harmful habits like smoking and excessive alcohol consumption. By fostering a healthier lifestyle, individuals can improve their digestive health and reduce the risk of diverticulitis flare-ups.

Integrative medicine plays a vital role in the treatment of diverticulosis and diverticulitis by offering a comprehensive, personalized approach that combines the best of conventional and complementary therapies. This holistic strategy not only addresses the immediate symptoms but also promotes overall health and well-being, helping individuals achieve long-term digestive health.

Mind-body connection and practices

The mind-body connection is a fundamental aspect of holistic health, emphasizing how mental and emotional states can significantly influence physical well-being. For individuals with diverticulosis and diverticulitis, understanding and nurturing this connection can be particularly beneficial. Mind-body practices can help manage stress, reduce inflammation, and improve overall digestive health.

1. Understanding the Mind-Body Connection:
The mind-body connection refers to the bidirectional relationship between our mental and emotional states and our physical health. Stress, anxiety, and other emotional factors can impact the digestive system, exacerbating symptoms of diverticulosis

and increasing the risk of diverticulitis flare-ups. Conversely, physical discomfort and chronic illness can affect mental health, creating a cycle of stress and illness.

2. Mindfulness and Meditation:
Mindfulness and meditation are powerful tools for enhancing the mind-body connection. These practices involve focusing attention on the present moment, often through breath awareness, body scanning, or guided imagery. Regular mindfulness practice can reduce stress and anxiety, lower cortisol levels, and promote relaxation. Meditation helps calm the nervous system, which can improve gut motility and reduce inflammation, benefiting those with digestive disorders.

3. Yoga:
Yoga combines physical postures, breath control, and meditation to promote physical and mental well-being. Specific yoga poses can stimulate the digestive system, enhance blood flow to the intestines, and relieve symptoms like bloating and constipation. Additionally, yoga's emphasis on deep breathing and relaxation helps reduce stress, which can positively impact digestive health.

4. Deep Breathing Exercises:
Deep breathing exercises, such as diaphragmatic breathing or pranayama, activate the body's relaxation response. By practicing deep breathing, individuals can lower their heart rate, reduce blood pressure, and promote a sense of calm. This can help mitigate the physical effects of stress on the digestive system, improving overall gut health.

5. Progressive Muscle Relaxation (PMR):
Progressive Muscle Relaxation involves systematically tensing and relaxing different muscle groups in the body. This practice can help individuals become more aware of physical tension associated with stress and learn to release it. PMR can reduce overall stress levels, improve sleep quality, and promote a sense of physical and mental relaxation, which benefits digestive health.

6. Tai Chi and Qigong:
Tai Chi and Qigong are ancient Chinese practices that combine gentle, flowing movements with breath control and meditation. These practices enhance the mind-body connection by promoting relaxation, reducing stress, and improving physical balance and flexibility. The slow, deliberate movements can

help stimulate digestive function and reduce symptoms related to digestive disorders.

7. Biofeedback:
Biofeedback is a technique that teaches individuals to control physiological functions by providing real-time feedback on bodily processes such as heart rate, muscle tension, and breathing. Through biofeedback, individuals can learn to manage stress responses more effectively, leading to improved digestive health and reduced symptoms of diverticulosis and diverticulitis.

8. Visualization and Guided Imagery:
Visualization and guided imagery involve creating mental images to promote relaxation and healing. These techniques can help reduce stress, lower anxiety, and enhance overall well-being. Guided imagery, in particular, can be used to visualize the digestive system functioning smoothly, which can have a positive impact on gut health.

By integrating mind-body practices into daily routines, individuals can strengthen the connection between their mental and physical health. These practices not only help manage stress and anxiety but also promote a more balanced and resilient digestive system. For those dealing with diverticulosis and diverticulitis, nurturing the mind-body connection can lead to significant improvements in symptoms and overall quality of life.

Acupuncture and other alternative therapies

Alternative therapies, including acupuncture, can play a valuable role in managing diverticulitis and diverticulosis. These therapies offer additional avenues for symptom relief, stress reduction, and overall improvement in digestive health. While they should complement, not replace, conventional medical treatments, many people find them beneficial in enhancing their overall wellness.

1. Acupuncture:
Acupuncture, a practice rooted in traditional Chinese medicine, involves the insertion of thin needles into specific points on the body to stimulate energy flow and promote healing. For individuals with diverticulitis and diverticulosis, acupuncture can help reduce pain, improve digestion, and decrease inflammation. Research suggests that acupuncture may regulate gut motility, enhance immune function,

and reduce stress, all of which are beneficial for managing digestive disorders.

2. Herbal Medicine:
Herbal remedies have been used for centuries to treat various ailments, including digestive issues. Herbs such as slippery elm, marshmallow root, and licorice root can soothe and protect the digestive tract, reduce inflammation, and promote healing. Additionally, anti-inflammatory herbs like turmeric and ginger can help manage symptoms of diverticulitis. It's important to consult with a healthcare provider before starting any herbal treatments to ensure they are safe and appropriate.

3. Probiotics:
Probiotics are beneficial bacteria that support gut health by maintaining a healthy balance of gut flora. These microorganisms can help reduce inflammation, improve bowel regularity, and enhance the overall function of the digestive system. Probiotic supplements or probiotic-rich foods, such as yogurt, kefir, sauerkraut, and kimchi, can be incorporated into the diet to support gut health.

4. Aromatherapy:

Aromatherapy uses essential oils extracted from plants to promote physical and emotional well-being. Essential oils like peppermint, ginger, and fennel can be particularly helpful for digestive health. Inhaling these oils or using them in a massage can help reduce symptoms such as bloating, gas, and abdominal discomfort. Aromatherapy also aids in stress reduction, which is beneficial for managing digestive conditions.

5. Chiropractic Care:
Chiropractic care involves the manipulation of the spine and other parts of the musculoskeletal system. This therapy can improve nervous system function, reduce pain, and enhance overall health. For individuals with digestive issues, chiropractic adjustments can help alleviate symptoms by improving nerve function related to the digestive organs and promoting better circulation and lymphatic flow.

6. Reflexology:
Reflexology is a practice that involves applying pressure to specific points on the feet, hands, or ears, which correspond to different organs and systems in the body. Reflexology can help stimulate digestive function, reduce stress, and promote

relaxation. Regular reflexology sessions can support overall digestive health and improve symptoms related to diverticulosis and diverticulitis.

7. Massage Therapy:
Massage therapy can be beneficial for managing stress and improving overall well-being. Techniques such as abdominal massage can help stimulate digestive function, relieve constipation, and reduce abdominal discomfort. General massage therapy also helps reduce stress and muscle tension, contributing to better digestive health.

8. Mindfulness-Based Stress Reduction (MBSR):
MBSR is a structured program that combines mindfulness meditation
and yoga to reduce stress and improve quality of life. Practicing mindfulness can help individuals become more aware of their stress triggers and manage their reactions, which is particularly useful for those with digestive disorders. MBSR programs have been shown to improve symptoms and enhance overall well-being in individuals with chronic illnesses.

Integrating these alternative therapies into a comprehensive treatment plan can provide additional support for individuals managing diverticulitis and diverticulosis. By addressing the physical, emotional, and psychological aspects of health, these therapies can contribute to a more holistic and effective approach to managing digestive conditions. Always consult with healthcare professionals to ensure that these therapies are safe and appropriate for your specific health needs.

Chapter 8

Living with Diverticulitis and Diverticulosis

Living with diverticulitis and diverticulosis can present unique challenges, but with the right knowledge, strategies, and support, individuals can lead healthy and fulfilling lives. This chapter focuses on practical advice, lifestyle adjustments, and emotional support necessary for managing these conditions on a day-to-day basis.

Understanding how to live with diverticulitis and diverticulosis involves more than just adhering to medical treatments; it requires a holistic approach that includes dietary modifications, regular physical activity, stress management, and regular medical monitoring. By integrating these elements into daily life, individuals can prevent flare-ups, manage symptoms effectively, and maintain overall digestive health.

In this chapter, we will explore various aspects of daily living with diverticulitis and diverticulosis.

Topics will include creating a supportive diet plan, incorporating regular exercise, utilizing stress management techniques, and navigating social and emotional aspects of living with a chronic digestive condition. Additionally, we will discuss how to work effectively with healthcare providers to ensure comprehensive care and address any concerns promptly.

The goal of this chapter is to empower individuals with practical tools and strategies to manage their condition proactively. By fostering a supportive and informed approach to living with diverticulitis and diverticulosis, individuals can improve their quality of life, reduce the frequency and severity of symptoms, and enjoy a greater sense of well-being.

Managing daily life with diverticular disease

Living with diverticular disease, which includes both diverticulosis and diverticulitis, requires ongoing attention to diet, lifestyle, and overall health management. By making thoughtful adjustments and adopting healthy habits, individuals can effectively manage their symptoms and reduce the risk of complications. Here are key strategies to help navigate daily life with diverticular disease:

1. Dietary Adjustments:
Maintaining a diet that supports digestive health is crucial. Focus on a high-fibre diet that includes plenty of fruits, vegetables, whole grains, and legumes. Fibre helps soften stool and promotes regular bowel movements, reducing the pressure on the colon that can lead to diverticula formation or inflammation. However, increase fibre intake gradually to prevent bloating and gas. Stay hydrated by drinking plenty of water throughout the day, as fibre works best when it absorbs water.

2. Eating Habits:
Adopt mindful eating habits to support digestive health. Eat smaller, more frequent meals rather than large ones, which can be easier on the digestive system. Chew food thoroughly to aid digestion and avoid rushing through meals. Additionally, avoid eating late at night to give your digestive system time to process food before bedtime.

3. Regular Physical Activity:
Incorporate regular exercise into your daily routine. Physical activity stimulates intestinal contractions,

promoting regular bowel movements and reducing the risk of constipation. Aim for at least 30 minutes of moderate exercise most days of the week. Activities such as walking, swimming, cycling, yoga, and strength training can be particularly beneficial.

4. Stress Management:
Chronic stress can negatively impact digestive health. Implementing stress management techniques can help alleviate symptoms and prevent flare-ups. Practices such as mindfulness meditation, deep breathing exercises, yoga, and tai chi can reduce stress and promote relaxation. Make time for hobbies and activities you enjoy to maintain a balanced lifestyle.

5. Avoiding Trigger Foods:
Identify and avoid foods that trigger symptoms. Common culprits include processed foods, red meat, high-fat foods, and foods that can cause gas or bloating. Keep a food diary to track what you eat and how it affects your symptoms, allowing you to make informed dietary choices.

6. Adequate Hydration:
Drinking plenty of water is essential for maintaining digestive health. Aim for at least eight 8-ounce

glasses of water daily. Proper hydration helps prevent constipation and supports the function of fibre in the diet.

7. Medication Management:
If prescribed, take medications as directed by your healthcare provider. This may include antibiotics for diverticulitis flare-ups or medications to manage symptoms such as pain or inflammation. Discuss any side effects or concerns with your doctor to ensure effective management of your condition.

8. Regular Medical Check-ups:
Stay proactive about your health by scheduling regular check-ups with your healthcare provider. Routine monitoring can detect any changes in your condition early and allow for timely intervention. Your doctor can also provide personalized advice on managing your symptoms and adjusting your treatment plan as needed.

9. Building a Support System:
Living with a chronic condition can be challenging, so it's important to build a support system. Connect with family and friends who understand your condition and can offer emotional support. Consider joining a support group, either in person or online, to

share experiences and gain insights from others living with diverticular disease.

10. Educating Yourself:
Stay informed about diverticular disease by reading reputable sources and discussing any questions or concerns with your healthcare provider.
Understanding your condition empowers you to make informed decisions about your health and manage your symptoms more effectively.

By incorporating these strategies into daily life, individuals with diverticular disease can manage their condition proactively, reduce symptoms, and improve their overall quality of life. Adopting a comprehensive approach that includes dietary changes, regular exercise, stress management, and ongoing medical care is key to living well with diverticular disease.

Coping strategies and support systems

Living with diverticular disease can be challenging, but adopting effective coping strategies and building a strong support system can significantly enhance quality of life. Here are some practical approaches to help manage the condition and find the necessary support:

1. Developing Coping Strategies:

a. Educate Yourself:
Knowledge is empowering. Understanding the nature of diverticular disease, its symptoms, triggers, and treatment options can help you make informed decisions about your health. Regularly consult reliable sources and keep abreast of new developments in managing the condition.

b. Maintain a Positive Outlook:
Focusing on the positive aspects of your life and what you can control can help manage the emotional impact of living with a chronic condition. Set realistic goals, celebrate small victories, and be patient with yourself during flare-ups or difficult times.

c. Practice Mindfulness and Relaxation Techniques:
Mindfulness meditation, deep breathing exercises, and progressive muscle relaxation can help reduce stress and improve your overall well-being. These techniques can be practiced daily and are

particularly helpful during periods of discomfort or stress.

d. Stay Organized:
Keep track of your symptoms, diet, and any medications you are taking. Maintaining a journal can help you identify patterns and triggers, which you can discuss with your healthcare provider to optimize your treatment plan.

e. Engage in Regular Physical Activity:
Exercise is beneficial for both physical and mental health. Activities like walking, swimming, yoga, and tai chi can improve your digestive health, reduce stress, and boost your mood.

f. Follow a Balanced Diet:
Adhering to a high-fibre diet, staying hydrated, and avoiding trigger foods can help manage symptoms. Work with a nutritionist if needed to develop a meal plan that suits your needs and preferences.

g. Prioritize Rest and Sleep:
Adequate rest and quality sleep are essential for healing and overall health. Establish a regular sleep routine and create a restful environment to promote better sleep.

2. Building a Support System:

a. Family and Friends:
Open communication with family and friends about your condition can foster understanding and support. Let them know how they can assist you, whether it's accompanying you to medical appointments, helping with daily tasks, or simply providing a listening ear.

b. Support Groups:
Joining a support group can provide a sense of community and shared understanding. These groups, either in-person or online, offer a platform to exchange experiences, coping strategies, and encouragement with others facing similar challenges.

c. Healthcare Team:
Building a strong relationship with your healthcare providers is crucial. Regular check-ups and open communication with your doctor, nutritionist, and other specialists ensure that your treatment plan is tailored to your needs and adjusted as necessary.

d. Counselling and Therapy:
Professional counselling or therapy can be beneficial for managing the emotional and psychological aspects of living with a chronic condition. Therapists can provide coping strategies, stress management techniques, and a safe space to express your feelings.

e. Online Communities and Resources:
Many online platforms and forums are dedicated to diverticular disease and digestive health. These communities offer valuable information, peer support, and a sense of connection to others who understand your journey.

f. Self-Help Resources:
Books, articles, podcasts, and videos on managing chronic illness can provide additional insights and motivation. Seek out resources that focus on holistic health, coping strategies, and personal stories of living with diverticular disease.

g. Social Activities and Hobbies:
Engaging in social activities and hobbies that you enjoy can provide a much-needed distraction and boost your mood. Whether it's reading, gardening, painting, or any other hobby, finding joy in these

activities can help reduce stress and improve overall well-being.

By combining effective coping strategies with a strong support system, individuals with diverticular disease can manage their condition more effectively and maintain a higher quality of life. The journey may have its challenges, but with the right tools and support, it is possible to lead a fulfilling and healthy life.

Conclusion

In conclusion, living with diverticulitis and diverticulosis presents unique challenges, but with the right knowledge, strategies, and support, individuals can lead healthy and fulfilling lives. This book has aimed to provide a comprehensive understanding of these conditions, from their causes and symptoms to various management and treatment options. By integrating conventional medical treatments with natural remedies, dietary modifications, and lifestyle changes, individuals can effectively manage their symptoms and prevent complications.

The importance of a holistic approach cannot be overstated. Addressing not only the physical aspects of diverticular disease but also the emotional and psychological components is crucial for overall well-being. Techniques such as mindfulness, meditation, yoga, and other stress-reduction practices play a significant role in managing this condition. Additionally, alternative therapies like acupuncture, herbal remedies, and probiotics offer complementary benefits that can enhance digestive health and alleviate symptoms.

Building a strong support system is another vital component of managing diverticular disease. Whether through family, friends, support groups, or healthcare professionals, having a network of support can make a significant difference in navigating the daily challenges of this condition. Open communication, education, and mutual understanding within this support system are key to fostering a positive and proactive approach to health.

It is essential to remember that every individual's journey with diverticulitis and diverticulosis is unique. Personalizing your management plan based on your specific needs, symptoms, and lifestyle is critical. Regular medical check-ups and ongoing dialogue with healthcare providers will ensure that your treatment plan remains effective and responsive to any changes in your condition.

As you move forward, continue to educate yourself about diverticular disease and stay informed about new research and treatments. Embrace the lifestyle changes and coping strategies that work best for you, and remain proactive in managing your health. By doing so, you can improve your quality of life, reduce the frequency and severity of flare-ups, and maintain better overall health.

Thank you for reading this book. It is my hope that the information and insights provided here will empower you to take control of your health and live well with diverticulitis and diverticulosis. Remember, you are not alone in this journey, and with the right tools and support, you can navigate this condition successfully and thrive.

Made in the USA
Monee, IL
11 August 2024